Clinical Supervision

Pacific
WITHDRAWN
University

Pacific
WITHDRAWN
University

For Churchill Livingstone:

Senior Commissioning Editor: Jacqueline Curthoys
Project Development Manager: Valerie Dearing
Project Manager: Derek Robertson

Clinical Supervision

A Practical Approach

Els van Ooijen MA BA(Hons) DipN DipCouns PGCE RGN RM

Lecturer, School of Nursing Studies
University of Wales College of Medicine
Caerleon, UK

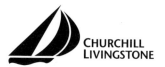

CHURCHILL
LIVINGSTONE

EDINBURGH LONDON NEW YORK PHILADELPHIA ST LOUIS SYDNEY
TORONTO 2000

PACIFIC UNIVERSITY LIBRARY
FOREST GROVE, OREGON

CHURCHILL LIVINGSTONE
An imprint of Harcourt Publishers Limited

© Harcourt Publishers Limited 2000

🖊 is a registered trademark of Harcourt Publishers Limited

The right of Els van Ooijen to be identified as author of this work has been
asserted by her in accordance with the Copyright, Designs and Patents Act 1988

All rights reserved. No part of this publication may be reproduced, stored in a
retrieval system, or transmitted in any form or by any means, electronic,
mechanical, photocopying, recording or otherwise, without either the prior
permission of the publishers (Harcourt Publishers Limited, 24–28 Oval Road,
London NW1 7DX), or a licence permitting restricted copying in the
United Kingdom issued by the Copyright Licensing Agency,
90 Tottenham Court Road, London W1P 0LP.

First published 2000

ISBN 0443 05842 3

British Library Cataloguing in Publication Data
A catalogue record for this book is available from the British Library

Library of Congress Cataloging in Publication Data
A catalog record for this book is available from the Library of Congress

The
publisher's
policy is to use
paper manufactured
from sustainable forests

Printed in China

3 5369 00269 8783

Contents

Acknowledgements

This idea for this book and the model discussed in Chapter 6 originated in conversations with my friend and fellow supervisor Patricia Osborne – thanks Tricia. My thanks are due also to all the people who have participated in the workshops, study days and courses I have held over the last six years and to those who have been (and continue to be) in supervision with me. I have learnt a great deal from all of you and hope to continue to do so for a very long time. The support of the people who found the time to try out the exercises, read the various drafts and help in various other ways has been invaluable and I am indebted to you all. Also, the supervision I have myself received, from Chris Evans, has been invaluable. Lastly, a big thank you to my partner Peter for his feedback on drafts of the manuscript and his continued support and encouragement.

Introduction

Much has happened since the publication of the position paper on clinical supervision by Butterworth & Faugier in 1994. From only very limited awareness initially, it is now unlikely that there are many nurses who have not heard about clinical supervision. As a lecturer in nurse education and a practising counsellor and supervisor, I have been running workshops and courses on supervision for a number of years now. What became clear to me initially was that there was widespread confusion about the nature and purpose of clinical supervision, coupled with a dearth of literature aimed specifically at nurses.

To date, the situation has not changed significantly. Although a vast amount of articles has appeared in recent years, there are few that deal with the nitty-gritty of what is involved. Also, the widespread confusion that exists is to some extent demonstrated by the very different views espoused. For example, some writers feel that supervision should be managerial and its implementation hierarchical, whereas others view that as anathema. I am aware that a managerial type of clinical supervision is implemented in other professions such as social work, but I feel that many of you will agree that the nursing culture is different and that a managerial approach to clinical supervision would meet with distrust, antagonism and resistance.

Most books on the subject deal mainly with supervision in counselling, psychotherapy and, occasionally, social work. There are still only a few publications aimed specifically at nurses, such as *Skills of Clinical Supervision* by Bond & Holland (1998) and a development pack published by the Open University (1998). I therefore decided to use my experience of practising and teaching supervision to write a book that discusses the practical aspects of the subject. In other words, this book is about 'What do I do?' and 'How do I do it?'. My aim is for you to feel that having read the book, you are clear on what it is all about, understand the skills needed, both for supervisors and supervisees, and will feel enthusiastic about getting involved.

I have deliberately not focused very much on the why and wherefore of clinical supervision as these are amply covered elsewhere. There is now a plethora of articles on the history and rationale for clinical supervision; a useful summary is also provided by Bond & Holland (1998).

WHO IS THIS BOOK WRITTEN FOR?

In a nutshell, everybody. Clinical supervision is not just for those at the bedside, but for all nurses regardless of their education, years of experience or area of work. Therefore, as supervision is for all nurses, so is this book. Perhaps you have been given the task of implementing clinical supervision in your area, or maybe you are interested in becoming a supervisor. Perhaps you would like to have supervision but want to know more before embarking on finding a supervisor. You may be a manager asked to evaluate the effectiveness of clinical supervision or an educationist charged with providing supervision training packages for any or all of the above. Whoever you are, this book is for you, as I have aimed to write a user-friendly book that is comprehensive while, at the same time, remaining practical. Although I have written it specifically for nurses, I feel that it is also relevant to those from other helping professions, such as occupational and physical therapy, speech therapy and social work as well as those involved with voluntary organisations. Basically, people from every occupation that is people-oriented and necessitates good interpersonal skills, including perhaps some counselling skills, may find this book useful, as I see supervision as helping people function to the best of their ability. This means that supervision is about every aspect of a person's job, not mainly about his or her work with particular clients, as is the case with counselling and psychotherapy, for example.

As far as nursing is concerned, traditionally, its unique culture has been rather defensive. Until relatively recently it was not acceptable for nurses to admit to feeling stressed or distressed about aspects of their work, and nurses did not feel comfortable in admitting to gaps in their knowledge, skills or experience. So although nursing is still a predominantly female occupation, these aspects of its culture seem curiously macho, which may be because it was originally modelled on the military.

These attitudes are beginning to change and nurses are now expected to provide more than just physical care for patients. However, in addition to becoming more involved with patients on an emotional and perhaps even spiritual level, more and more is included in a nurse's work, such as quality assurance and budgeting as well as tasks previously thought to be the province of our medical colleagues. At the same time, an effect of the internal market has been the importance of efficiency as well as the need to provide a cost-effective service, which often meant a reduction in the numbers and calibre of staff.

Faced with all these stresses, nurses need the time and space to reflect on what is happening and what all this means for them, their work and the patients for whom they care. Supervision in nursing therefore gives practitioners an opportunity to reflect on all aspects of their work, as ultimately everything they do will have an effect on the care that patients receive.

HOW TO USE THIS BOOK

I refer in the above heading to you 'using' the book, not just reading it, which means engaging with it, thinking about the material and agreeing or disagreeing with it. In fact, you should read it with irreverence, highlight passages that make an impact, write in the margins where it makes you think; in short, personalise it and make it a working guide for you. While reading the chapters on the supervisory relationship and the development of supervisees and supervisors (Chapters 2–5), it is recommended that you keep a reflective journal in which to complete the activities suggested. I urge you to do so as the more you engage with the book, the more you are likely to gain from it.

Although there is a clear sequence to its structure, you do not necessarily have to start at the beginning, but may prefer to dip into a chapter in which you have a particular interest. Chapter 1 provides an overview of some of the better-known supervision models. Most of these originate from outside the profession but can be adapted to the nursing situation, although their suitability will depend on the area of nursing involved. This is the most theoretical part of the book. However, if you would rather start with the practice rather than the theory you may like to read it last.

The remainder of the book deals with the nitty-gritty of supervision and all that is involved. In Chapter 2, the importance of a good supervisory relationship is discussed, as well as choosing a supervisor who is right for you and negotiating a clear and useful contract. Chapter 3 deals with the preparation and development of necessary skills for supervisees, whereas in Chapter 4, the emphasis is on the skills needed for supervisors. In chapter 5, I introduce my Double Helix Model of Supervisory Development, which I see as a useful framework for the preparation and development of supervisors. Chapter 6 is the largest chapter of the book as here I discuss the entire phenomenon of clinical supervision in light of the Double Helix Model. I aim to answer questions such as 'What do I actually do?', 'How can I help people really reflect rather than skim the surface?', or even 'How do I help people to achieve that "super" vision?'. The bulk of this chapter therefore deals with the process of clinical supervision in the form of scenarios which are then discussed in light of the Double Helix Model. I should point out here that the model was developed in close collaboration with my friend and fellow supervisor/lecturer, Patricia Osborne, with whom I have done much work over the past few years. The model is therefore based on our practice of supervising individuals and groups, as well as our experience of running many workshops on the subject. I see the strength of the model in that it has been developed specifically for the nursing profession. The case scenarios that appear here, as well as elsewhere in the book, are based on my own experience, but in order to maintain confidentiality, I have engaged in a certain amount of mixing and matching. Every scenario is therefore an amalgam of different people and situations, which means that it will not be possible for individual people to be identifiable. In order to avoid any gender bias, I have used the pronouns 'he' and 'she' interchangeably throughout the book.

Finally, all I want to say is that I hope that you will enjoy using this book as much as I have enjoyed writing it.

REFERENCES

Bond M, Holland S 1998 Skills of clinical supervision. Open University Press Milton Keynes
Butterworth T, Faugier J 1994 Clinical supervision in nursing, midwifery and health visiting: a briefing paper. School of Nursing Studies, University of Manchester
Open University 1998 Clinical supervision: a development pack for nurses. K509. Open University Press, Milton Keynes

Models of supervision

Supervision is much more complex than I at first imagined. (Carroll 1996: 3)

Nursing is essentially a practical discipline and clinical supervision is concerned with maintaining and improving that practice. Supervision is therefore about functioning effectively, whenever and wherever. So the focus of the supervision needs to be the nurse–patient interaction, but it could also usefully involve interactions between the nurse and other members of the health care team, as ultimately, these will have an effect on the patients. Through the reflection that takes place in supervision, nurses are able to look at their practice in a different way, helping them to make it truly reflective.

MODELS OF SUPERVISION

In this chapter, the more prevalent models of supervision are classified according to theoretical background or function, followed by a more detailed discussion of those models most likely to be useful to nursing.

CLASSIFICATION

Whereas, traditionally, supervision formed part of the process of becoming a professional therapist, counsellor or social worker, increasingly supervision is being seen as a discipline in its own right. So although supervision courses still tend to attract mainly counsellors and psychotherapists, there is a growing representation from other disciplines such as social work, art therapy or nursing in learning about supervision itself.

With perhaps the exception of Johns' Reflective Cycle (Johns 1997), most of the theories and models of supervision have been developed within the areas of psychotherapy, counselling and social work. It would therefore be inadvisable to apply them uncritically and altered for nursing without testing their effectiveness and appropriateness. Indeed there is currently some debate within these disciplines as to whether or not models developed in one area of, say, psychotherapy are applicable to another. This is in line with the view that as far as nursing is concerned, models of supervision need to be specific to be useful, as they may not be transferable between different health care settings (Smith 1995, Butterworth et al 1996).

It seems that the more practical a model is, the more possible it is to use it across disciplines. However, choice of an appropriate model is clearly important (Faugier 1994 in Smith 1995). Whereas most of the models discussed in this chapter would seem to be applicable, to a greater or lesser degree, across settings, those which rely on a particular psychotherapeutic theory (so-called 'approach-bound' models) may not be appropriate for use outside the mental health arena. In this context, it seems to me that some of the approach-bound models might be usefully combined with a pure supervision model. In other words, the supervision model might provide the structure, the actual approach influencing the process.

Research in supervision has tended to focus on a particular model or way of working rather than on comparing models for content, efficacy or relevance to context. Also, much research that does exist has been carried out in the USA and at present, it is not clear to what extent findings and conclusions are applicable to the UK (Carroll 1996: 9). This is because in the USA, the main approach of supervision has been developmental (Hawkins & Shohet 1989: 48), with its focus being largely conceptual and intellectual. In the UK, on the other hand, emphasis has been much more on practice and training (Carroll 1996: 18), with a more eclectic approach to usage of models. However, even in the USA, supervision was not recognised as a practice distinct from counselling or therapy until the 1980s (Holloway 1995: xi).

DEVELOPMENTAL MODELS

Developmental models are derived from developmental psychology and emphasise primarily the educational function of supervision. As nurses may vary in their levels of knowledge or experience, familiarity with a developmental model is useful. Indeed, a developmental model may be integrated with a more supervision-focused model. In psychotherapy and social work, supervision is to a large extent associated with training and education, and it may well be that in time, developmental supervision will form an important aspect of pre-registration nurse education.

According to Holloway, 18 different developmental models can be found in the literature (Holloway 1995: 4). Hawkins & Shohet mention a number of developmental models (Hogan 1964, Worthington 1987, Stoltenberg & Delworth 1987) which they then go on to integrate into a 'combined developmental model of four major stages of supervisee development' (Hawkins & Shohet 1989: 49). Regarding nursing, Benner's (1984) view of the nurse as moving from novice to expert is now widely adopted.

The following discussion of developmental models is partly based on Hawkins & Shohet's explanation and applied to the nursing situation.

Level 1 (child, novice)

Although highly motivated, at level 1, the supervisee lacks insight and has not yet developed an overview of the therapeutic process. She is likely to feel insecure which leads her to be dependent on her supervisor. As she has not yet developed grounded criteria, it is difficult for her to assess her own performance. Part of becoming a proficient worker involves being able to reflect, to develop an 'internal supervisor' as it were. At this level, however, the nurse's internal supervisor is still immature. There is also a tendency to jump to premature conclusions without sufficient information.

The task of the supervisor at this level is to provide a structured environment and positive feedback. In other words, supervisees need a great deal of encouragement and recognition for the work that they are doing, while being helped to reflect in a systematic way.

Level 2 (adolescent, journeyman)

At this level, the supervisee has a tendency to swing from dependence to autonomy and from feeling overwhelmed to feeling overconfident. At level 2, the nurse becomes aware that there is more to nursing than initially thought. She may realise that the 'art' of nursing can be tricky and elusive, yet terribly important and that the science of nursing is arid without the art. The supervisee may also realise that there is more to nursing than learning all the theories, skills and procedures. When things go well, she may feel overconfident, only to crash to self-doubt when something goes wrong. Like adolescence, this can be a difficult and stormy stage, the fluctuations in confidence, independence and security leading to a sense of insecurity and fear, which may be vented on the supervisor in the form of anger. In the same way that adolescents may rebel against their parents and attack them (indeed this is for many people a necessary stage), the supervisee at level 2 may argue with the supervisor and question his views and competence.

The supervisor needs to be able to provide an environment where it is possible for the supervisee to express negative emotions, and the supervisor also needs to know when to support and when to let go, which will inevitably mean taking risks. This requires good facilitative skills and a level of maturity. It would be unhelpful for the supervisor to be caught up in the supervisee's maturational process and to become defensive or punitive under attack.

This level can occur during the second year of pre-registration training, but often resurfaces later when additional, perhaps threatening, skills or education (such as supervision) are taken on. Interestingly, level 2-type antagonism is frequently encountered in training for clinical supervision. During the level 1 phase of training, nurses are interested and may see it as a good idea. However, as they learn more about what is actually involved, they may become insecure regarding their own competence or ability to develop the skills required. Thus they may either reject supervision altogether as an unrealistic idea, say it is not needed because 'we already do it unofficially anyway', or doubt the organisation's willingness to provide sufficient support (even if the organisation is committed to its implementation and is investing money into training).

Level 3 (young adulthood, independent craftsman)

Levels of security and confidence no longer fluctuate dramatically, as the nurse becomes increasingly able to trust her own judgement and competence. The relationship with the supervisor becomes more colleagial, and when disagreements do occur, they are like professional discussions about different viewpoints rather than personal attacks.

Hawkins & Shohet (1989: 51) mention that a person at this stage has developed the ability to function at various levels simultaneously. For example, while seeing to a patient's immediate needs, the nurse will also be mindful of his personal life circumstances and how they are affected by his illness, the relationship she has built up with the patient in the context in which she works, as well as how both she and the patient are affected by and in turn can affect, that context. In other words, rather than only focusing on the physical and the here and now, the nurse is able simultaneously to be aware of the totality of the situation in a holistic way. At this stage, the supervisor needs to pull back and trust the nurse's development, providing support, guidance or challenge where appropriate.

Level 4 (mature adult, master craftsman, expert)

At this level the nurse feels secure in her own capabilities and trusts her own judgement. She is able to function autonomously, while at the same time recognising the limits of that autonomy within an environment where teamwork is essential. Others are likely to recognise her ability and maturity and turn to her for advice, guidance and support.

A nurse at level 4 has developed a great deal of self-awareness, which, paradoxically, also means that she is aware of her limitations, as well as of the need to continue to reflect, learn and develop, as there is never a point at which development stops. So this is a stage of deepening and integration, rather than of acquiring more knowledge, of lighting the candle of wisdom (Hawkins & Shohet 1989: 52).

A major disadvantage of developmental models is that their usefulness decreases linearly as the surpervisee becomes more experienced. They are therefore not likely to be suitable for experienced nurses, unless they are in an environment or learning situation that is new to them. Another limitation is that although developmental models outline the stages of supervisees' development, they do not provide an explanation of *how* change occurs in either the supervisee or the supervisor, and there appears to be a distinct paucity in relevant research (Carroll 1996: 16).

APPROACH-BOUND MODELS

As supervision originally developed as part of counsellor or therapist training, the way in which it was practised tended to be according to the particular therapeutic approach on which the training was based. In other words, supervision was largely 'approach-bound'. Supervision as part of a person-centred training would therefore be person-centred, whereas someone learning to become a cognitive therapist would receive cognitive supervision.

An advantage of approach-bound supervision is that the supervisee, in addition to practising the approach, is also at the receiving end of it, the supervisor acting as a role model. A disadvantage is that with this type of supervision, the boundaries between supervision and counselling or therapy may become blurred, which is likely to lead to dissatisfaction. The issue of boundaries will be discussed further in the section on contracting in Chapter 2. Also, interventions that are useful in one arena are often not appropriate in another. Increasingly it is argued that supervision, as it is a separate activity with different purposes, goals and functions, requires models and skills other than those used in counselling, therapy or other helping professions.

However, as supervision develops, it is likely that people will develop their own ways of working, which may well be a synthesis of a number of models. It seems useful, for example, to always be aware of the developmental model, as it is obviously important to match the supervision to the developmental level of the supervisee. It would be pointless, indeed annoying, for example, to provide level 1-type supervision for a nurse who had reached the level of expert in her development. Conversely, to treat a nurse at level 2 as if she were an expert would be experienced as unsupportive and frightening by the supervisee, and could even be dangerous if inappropriate practice is not identified.

STRUCTURAL MODELS

The cyclical model

The Cyclical Model forms a comprehensive framework for the whole of supervision. It provides a step-by-step guide as to what to do, starting from the first meeting between potential supervisor and supervisee. As such it is very useful, both for teaching supervision and as a blueprint for when people first start out.

As Page & Wosket point out, a model is concerned both with structure and process, with the 'what' and the 'how' of supervision (Page & Wosket 1994: 29). The Cyclical Model was developed for use in counselling but lends itself easily to adaptation for use in the nursing context as the structure is reminiscent of other frameworks already familiar to nurses, such as the nursing process or the audit cycle.

Figure 1.1 represents a diagram of a supervision session in five stages. Although it appears to start with contract and end with review, its cyclical structure means that supervision can be started at any stage, depending on the needs of the supervisee and the situation. Each stage encompasses a number of issues, concepts and processes.

Stage 1: Contract (ground rules, boundaries, accountability, expectations, relationship)

As will be seen in Chapter 2, regardless of the model used, before two or more people decide to start a supervisory relationship, they will need to discuss a contract, so that those concerned know where they are. In other words, supervisor and supervisee will between them set the ground rules and boundaries, decide who

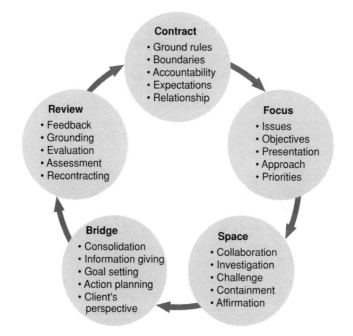

Figure 1.1   Cyclical Model (adapted from Page & Wosket 1994).

is accountable for what, and discuss any expectations that both have of the process and what type of relationship is preferred. However, contracting is not a once-and-for-all event, as contracts may be amended or renegotiated as the relationship develops and also as a result of the evaluation that takes place in the Review stage. For a further discussion of contracting see Chapter 2.

Stage 2: Focus (issue, objectives, presentation, approach, priorities)

In order to use the supervision well, it is important that any topic for discussion is agreed upon; however, sometimes a supervisee may be quite vague regarding the issue and need help to focus on a specific angle or angles. Having agreed what to focus on, it is important to stick to this and not to veer from it prematurely, before the issue has been reflected on satisfactorily and possible action planned.

Having agreed an issue, it is useful to clarify objectives, so that both supervisor and supervisee know what the purpose of bringing the issue to supervision is. Having clear objectives also makes the evaluation of the session in the Review stage easier, and can even form the basis for a more formal organisational review.

How an issue or topic is presented may be agreed in the contract. For example, some supervisors working in mental health find it helpful to read case notes, a reflective journal or a summary of the issue, topic or problem, whereas others prefer a verbal presentation. Whatever method of presentation is preferred, it is helpful for the supervisee to reflect on what she is bringing prior to the session.

Stage 3: Space (collaboration, investigation, challenge, containment, affirmation)

This stage is described as 'the heart of the supervision process' (Page & Wosket 1994: 35) and indeed, it is this stage that is the main focus of process-oriented models such as the Double Matrix Model. The Space stage is characterised by a tolerance of confusion and not knowing and commitment to exploration, which may at times be quite challenging for the supervisee. 'Challenge', as Page & Wosket (1994: 109) point out 'is strong medicine and should only be administered in small doses'. Even the question 'Tell me, what was your reason for doing *x*?' can be experienced as implied criticism. The relationship between supervisor and supervisee needs therefore to be collaborative and supportive with the nature of a 'reflective alliance' (Page & Wosket 1994: 99). Such a reflective alliance provides a space for both supervisee and supervisor to reflect on the issue brought as well as on the supervision process itself.

Stage 4: Bridge (consolidation, information giving, goal setting, action planning, client's perspective)

Having reflected thoroughly on an issue, the clearer perspective or 'super' vision is consolidated by, for example, the supervisor asking 'how do you see things now?', perhaps followed by 'what do you want to do with it?' It is at this stage that the supervisor may give relevant knowledge or experience if it seems useful. She may recommend a book or mention a study day she has heard about, for example, or share what happened in a similar situation. This should not be confused with advice; it is merely a sharing of information which the supervisee may or may not decide to use. Having consolidated the reflection and discussed relevant information, the supervisee may like to set goals and plan action, while considering what effect such action will have on others concerned (client's perspective).

Stage 5: Review (feedback, grounding, evaluation, assessment, recontracting)

It is useful to set aside time at the end of each supervision to evaluate the session itself, in order to see what worked, what did not and how useful the session was overall. In addition, it is good practice to build into the contract, regular reviews of the whole process say, every 6 months.

Johns' Reflective Cycle

Page & Wosket's Cyclical Model is not unlike Johns' Reflective Cycle, which has been specifically developed for use in the nursing context and, in its latest version, is also influenced by the work of Carper (Carper 1978, Johns 1997; see Fig. 1.2).

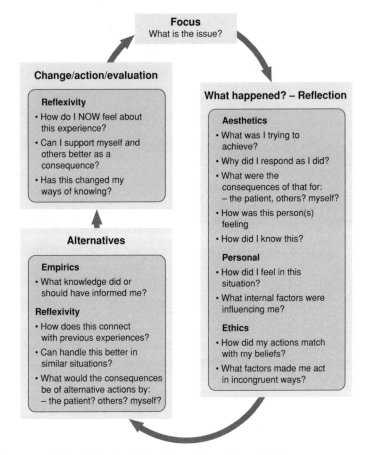

Figure 1.2 The Reflective Cycle (adapted from Johns 1997).

As can be seen from Figure 1.2, the cycle starts with 'what is the issue?' which is similar to the Focus stage in the Cyclical Model. The cycle then focuses on the facts (what happened) followed by a further reflection on those facts. It seems that this stage of the cycle would fit neatly within the Space section of the cyclical model, with the cycle's next two stages, which deal with alternative actions, their consequences and desired outcomes, appearing similar to the Bridge stage. So it could be argued that Johns' Reflective Cycle is not unlike Page & Wosket's Cyclical Model of supervision but without the Contract and Review stages.

The Matrix Model

Although the Matrix Model provides a clear structure of supervision, its approach is also developmental, which is how supervision has mainly been regarded in the USA (Hawkins & Shohet 1989: 48). In her book *Clinical Supervision: A Systems Approach*, Holloway (1995) states that the goal of supervision is to connect theory and practice (p. iii) in a spirit of 'meaningful empiricism' (p. xiv). The model has been developed to meet four needs:

a. a descriptive base
b. guidelines stating common goals and imperatives
c. a way to discover meaning as it relates to participants and the profession
d. a systematic mode of inquiry to determine objectives and strategies for interaction during supervision. (Holloway 1995: 5)

and is described as a 'heuristic tool to incorporate three sources of knowledge – theory, research and practice' (p. 6).

As may be seen in Figure 1.3, the supervision relationship is regarded as the core to the model and is placed centrally, with the other six dimensions coming out as wings at the side. The relationship between the seven dimensions is dynamic, with each dimension influencing and being influenced by the six others.

The two bottom wings, tasks and functions, represent the process of supervision, as illustrated in Figure 1.4. The model was developed for use in counselling training, hence the task 'counselling skill'; in the nursing context this could translate as interpersonal skills with patients, relatives, colleagues and others in the multidisciplinary team. The developmental nature of the model is evident in the function 'advising/instructing' which does not

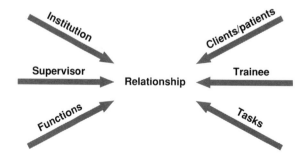

Figure 1.3   The Matrix Model (adapted from Holloway 1995).

appear appropriate in the professional supervision of qualified nurses, but could be relevant if supervision became part of pre-registration preparation.

Tasks

Case conceptualisation in the counselling context means the supervisor and supervisee working to understand each client's psychosocial history and current issues, in light of relevant theory. As such, it would be useful in the psychiatric context, or indeed whenever a nurse is working with someone in a psychological way, such as perhaps in bereavement, rehabilitation or oncology.

Professional role is about working professionally, according to the UKCC Code of Conduct (United Kingdom Central Council for Nursing, Midwifery and Health Visiting 1992) and the policies of the organisation as well as the nurse's own professional judgement, using whatever appropriate resources are available. Holloway also includes in this task, record keeping and participation in the supervisory relationship.

Emotional awareness is similar to parts of the 'what happened' section of Johns' Reflective Cycle (Johns, 1997) and refers to awareness of both the nurse's own feelings and emotions and those of others, be they patients, relatives or team members. Like Page & Wosket, Holloway refers to the usefulness of 'parallel process' as a vehicle for becoming aware of unconscious processes (see the Double Matrix Model, p. 18).

Self-evaluation is an accepted part of counselling education, where trainees are asked to reflect honestly on their performance with a particular client. Except perhaps in mental health, we have not traditionally employed self-evaluation in nursing, perhaps because admitting to not being totally perfect every time is

Tasks	Functions
• Counselling skill	• Monitoring/evaluating
• Case conceptualisation	• Advising/instructing
• Professional role	• Modelling
• Emotional awareness	• Consulting
• Self evaluation	• Supporting/sharing

Figure 1.4 The Matrix Model (adapted from Holloway 1995).

regarded as risky and possibly not without repercussions. If supervision is taken on board, then this type of honest self-evaluation is crucial and may be a sign that we are beginning to mature as a profession (van Ooijen 1994).

Functions

The functions are basically the activities engaged in by the supervisor and appear self-explanatory. The skills and tasks of the supervisor will be discussed in more detail in Chapter 3.

As seen above, Holloway states that 'tasks and functions = process' (p. 37). In other words, together they form the way in which supervisor and supervisee work together and influence each other. The other parts of the model relate to the context in which supervision takes place (that of the institution, the clients seen, the supervisor and the supervisee) and the supervisory relationship. Recognising the importance of contextual factors is useful, particularly to nursing as very few nurses work in isolation, but are part of a team within a larger organisation. In other words, the way in which a ward, unit or trust is organised may affect how individual nurses work with patients. If workloads are high, for example, perhaps through 'compassion fatigue', leading to disengagement, rather than seeing people as individuals, a nurse in this position may relate to patients as objects and reduce her care to the physical only (Jackson et al 1986 in Holloway 1995: 100), a process well documented by Menzies Lyth (1988).

Whereas all other functions are either structural (tasks and functions), or contextual, it is through the relationship that the supervision takes place, which is why Holloway has placed it at the core of the model and refers to it as 'the dynamic element of supervision' (Holloway 1995: 41). I agree with Holloway's view which is why I have devoted the next chapter to it, in which the relationship section of her model will be discussed in more detail (see Chapter 2).

PROCESS MODELS

The Double Matrix Model

Although a useful working model, the Double Matrix Model is concerned with only part of the supervision process, and does not really address contextual or organisational factors. On examination, the Double Matrix Model appears to cover the Tasks and Functions parts of Holloway's model and could be said to fit in the Space, and perhaps part of the Bridge sections of the Cyclical Model, or the second, third and fourth sections of Johns' Reflective Cycle.

The model (see Fig. 1.5) consists of two overlapping circles or matrixes which represent the client – nurse relationship (the therapy matrix) and the supervisee–supervisor relationship (the supervision matrix). Each matrix may be further subdivided into three categories, resulting in a total of six modes of supervision. The two circles are interlocked, the crucial person being the

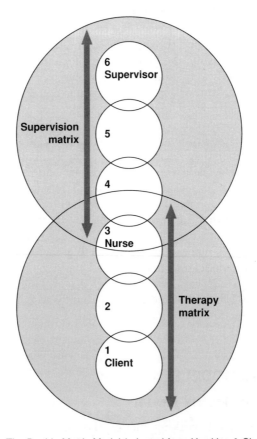

Figure 1.5 The Double Matrix Model (adapted from Hawkins & Shohet 1989).

supervisee. The task of the supervisor is to 'pay attention to' the therapy matrix; however, the way in which this is done will depend on the style of the supervisor. Broadly speaking, there are two main styles: in the first, supervisor and supervisee reflect together on the work done with the patient (modes 1, 2 and 3), whereas in the second style, the supervisor uses the here and now of the supervision session to reflect on the therapy matrix (modes 4, 5 and 6) (Hawkins & Shohet 1989: 56). According to Hawkins & Shohet, their model can be usefully combined with a developmental approach, moving from mode 1 towards mode 6 as supervisees get more experienced (p. 73). Although supervisors differ as to which style they prefer, good supervision, according to Hawkins & Shohet, should move between all modes, although not every mode needs to be addressed in every session (P. 72).

The Double Matrix Model is a useful working model, but can be difficult to comprehend. In my experience it is therefore best understood by experiential learning methods or by being at the receiving end of this type of supervision.

The Seven Tasks of Supervision Model

Like the Double Matrix Model, the Seven Tasks Model focuses on the process of supervision and is based on research which involved interviewing supervisors concerned with understanding what supervision is about. In the book *Counselling Supervision: Theory, Skills and Practice*, Carroll (1996) describes the model as a series of frameworks. In other words, it is basically an explanation of the supervision process and focuses on seven generic, summative or foundation tasks which pertain across models. Although the model is primarily developmental, it can also be used by experienced supervisors. Briefly, the Seven Tasks or 'Linear' Model connects the goals, functions and tasks of supervision (Carroll 1996: 17). The seven tasks appear to be a more comprehensive version of Proctor's three functions of supervision (Proctor, 1988) and include:

- to create the learning relationship
- to teach
- to counsel
- to consult
- to evaluate
- to monitor professional/ethical issues

- to work with the administrative/organisational aspects of client work (Carroll 1996: 16–17).

Although useful in describing the tasks a supervisor has to address, for nursing, the model appears less helpful than the Double Matrix Model in that it addresses the 'what', but not really the 'how' of supervision. However, Carroll's model may be useful as an evaluation tool for supervisors to check their own performance.

Whereas most tasks are self-explanatory, the task 'to counsel' is open to confusion, particularly as the British Association for Counselling (BAC) has drawn a distinct line between counselling and supervision and has stated that on no account can one function as counsellor and supervisor for the same person (BAC 1996). Carroll (1996) points out that the counselling task of supervision, referred to as 'helping supervisees reflect on any personal reactions arising out of working with clients', is distinct from personal counselling or therapy (p. 59), the difference being in the aims of the activity. He states 'The aim of supervision is to help supervisees become better workers, whereas the aim of counselling stresses becoming a better person' (p. 59). Leaving aside whether one agrees with this definition of counselling, it may be less confusing to use the word 'support' rather than counsel, especially as this is one of the functions identified by Proctor (1988) and Kadushin (1992), but which is absent from the Seven Tasks.

To be fair, it should be pointed out that Carroll's model is based on his research, which despite the BAC's stance, indicates some differences of opinion regarding the extent to which supervisors are prepared to let supervisees work on their own issues. There did, however, appear to be a consensus that only those personal issues arising from client work are legitimate topics for supervision.

DISCIPLINE-SPECIFIC MODELS

The models discussed thus far have mostly originated from the counselling/therapy arena, taking either a developmental stance, focusing on a particular theoretical approach, or one based on the structure or process of supervision. Whereas the use of approach-bound supervision models is likely to be limited outside mental health nursing, it seems that the other types of supervision models may usefully be adapted to other helping professions. At the same time, it is recognised that although all helping professionals work with people, how they carry out their work, and in what context, varies greatly. Thus, models of supervision pertaining to a specific discipline are beginning to be developed. Brown & Bourne (1996) describe their model developed for social work supervision as a 'map of the terrain' rather than as a prescription (p. 66). As such, it is intended as a tool to be used in whatever way people find useful. The model takes cognisance of the fact that, unlike many counsellors, social workers do not work in isolation, but are part of a larger system. Consequently, Brown & Bourne base their model on four systems: the practice system; the worker system; the team system; and the agency system (Brown & Bourne 1996: 67; Fig. 1.6).

'Practice' refers to the people social workers work with, who Brown & Bourne are reluctant to call 'clients' as many do not choose to be worked with and may indeed be at the receiving end of some unpleasant social work decisions. Examples of such decisions include having one's benefit refused, or a child taken into care. As Brown & Bourne (1996) rightly state, 'to call the recipients of these alleged services "clients" only adds insult to injury' (p. 68). Except perhaps in health education and preventative work, there are clear similarities between the social work practice system and nursing practice. Most people do not choose to be patients and would prefer not to be in need of medical or nursing care. The other systems appear equally applicable to nursing, 'team' refers

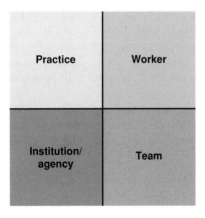

Figure 1.6   A model developed for social work supervision (adapted from Brown & Bourne 1996).

to colleagues, 'worker' to the supervisee and her resources, and 'agency' to the employing organisation, which includes any 'codes of practice, policies, procedures and guidelines' (Brown & Bourne 1996: 68).

In social work, supervision is often part of training, which is why Brown & Bourne (1996) suggest that supervisory development happens in three phases: induction, connection and integration, respectively. It is envisaged that in the induction phase, people work with each of the four systems fairly discretely, beginning to see connections in the next phase but fully integrating them in the integrative phase. It is this last phase that is the focus of super-vision with experienced workers and which may also include longer-term considerations, such as career planning (Brown & Bourne 1996: 73). In the integrative phase, the supervisee may well be more expert in her particular field than the supervisor; a main concern is therefore the prevention of stagnation by providing 'a sense of challenge' and the nurturing of creativity (p. 73). Such supervision would seem relevant for many nurses and might usefully take the form of peer consultancy.

CONCLUSION

In this chapter, I have discussed those supervisory models most likely to be helpful to nursing. From the discussion it is clear that there is a certain amount of overlap between models, and that the most useful models will probably integrate various uses and functions. Hawkins & Shohet's model, for example, is described as a process model in that it focuses on what actually happens during supervision; however, it may also be used as part of a developmental approach. As far as nursing is concerned, there is unlikely to be one model that fits all as there are so many different areas and activities in nursing. However, in Chapter 6 we intro-duce a model that has been developed specifically for nursing and which takes into account the unique features of nursing as well as the context of health care in which it takes place.

REFERENCES

British Association for Counselling 1996 Code of ethics and practice for supervisors of counsellors. BAC, Rugby

Benner P 1984 From novice to expert. Addison-Wesley, Menlo Park, CA

Brown A, Bourne I 1996 The social work supervisor. Open University Press, Buckingham

Butterworth T, Bishop V, Carson J 1996 First steps towards evaluating clinical supervision in nursing and health visiting. I. Theory, policy and practice development. A review. Journal of Clinical Nursing 5: 127–132

Carper B A 1978 Fundamental patterns of knowing in nursing. Advances in Nursing Science 1: 13–23

Carroll M 1996 Counselling supervision. Theory, skills and practice. Cassell, London

Hawkins P, Shohet R 1989 Supervision in the helping professions. Open University Press, Buckingham

Hogan R A 1964 Issues and approaches in supervision. Psychotherapy: Theory, Research and Practice 1: 139–141

Holloway E 1995 Clinical supervision. A systems approach. Sage, London

Johns C 1997 Reflective practice and clinical supervision – part I: the reflective turn. European Nurse 2(2): 87–97

Kadushin A 1992 Supervision in social work, 3rd edn. Columbia University Press, New York

Menzies Lyth E E P 1988 The functioning of social systems as a defence against anxiety: a report on a study of the nursing service of a general hospital. In: Menzies Lyth I. Containing anxiety in institutions. Free Association Books, London, p 43–85

Page S, Wosket V 1994 Supervising the counsellor. A cyclical model. Routledge, London

Polanyi M 1969 Knowing and being. University of Chicago, Illinois

Proctor B 1988 Supervision: a working alliance. Alexia, Sussex

Smith J P 1995 Clinical supervision: conference organised by the National Health Service Executive on 29 November 1994 at the National Motorcycle Museum, Solihull, West Midlands, England. Conference Report. Journal of Advanced Nursing 21: 1029–1031

Stoltenberg C D, Delworth V 1987 Supervising counselors and therapists. Josey Bass, San Francisco

United Kingdom Central Council for Nursing, Midwifery and Health Visiting 1992 Code of Conduct for the Nurse, Midwife and Health Visitor. UKCC, London

van Ooijen E G 1994 Whipping up a storm. Nursing Standard 9(8): 48

Worthington E L 1987 Changes in supervision as counselors and supervisors gain experience: a review. Professional Psychology: Research and Practice 18(3): 189–208

2

The supervisory relationship

A good working relationship is at the heart of effective supervision.

The supervisory relationship is the means by which other relationships (with patients, clients, relatives, colleagues, doctors, managers) are reflected upon and analysed, and through which learning takes place. In fact it may be seen as a 'microcosm of the wider society' (Brown & Bourne 1996: 82).

The Double Helix Model in particular makes use of the relationship to enhance awareness (see Chapter 6). This awareness may occur at two levels. First, giving attention to what is happening in the relationship between supervisor and supervisee can often reflect aspects of the situation under discussion. Second, attending to the way in which the supervisory relationship develops provides an opportunity to reflect on how both parties tend to begin and develop relationships in general. None of us is a blank slate and in meeting new people we inevitably bring with us our personal history, conceptions, misconceptions, experiences and prejudices. If, for example, because of an unpleasant past experience, a nurse has a problem with authority, this may unwittingly result in hostile and withholding behaviour towards the supervisor. This can happen even if the nurse has actually taken the initiative and selected the supervisor, as these types of problems are not always within our immediate conscious awareness.

This chapter is in four parts. In the first section, I discuss the issue of choice; in the second, the topic of power is discussed, followed by the development of the relationship in the third section, which includes an account of what is involved in contracting. Finally, in the last section, specific issues, learning opportunities and possible problems are discussed by means of examples and scenarios.

CHOICE

Managerial or consultative supervision?

Choice and self-determination have been described as the 'bottom line' of professional development (Barker 1996). Choices to be made include the type of supervision, who chooses whom and the framework or model to be used. As discussed in Chapter 1, there appears to be a difference between this country and the USA, where supervision is mostly carried out as part of training and is therefore largely developmental. Although supervision as part of training may be a useful idea to adopt in pre-registration nursing, this is not yet happening in the UK and most of the literature regarding supervision in the nursing press refers to the supervision of people post-registration.

For qualified practitioners, the choice is between consultative or managerial supervision. In consultative supervision, the supervisor does not have any managerial responsibility for the supervisee and might therefore work in a completely different area, for a different employer or even privately. Managerial supervision, on the other hand, is carried out either by the supervisee's manager, or by a person in the organisation who is expected to report back to the manager on how the supervisee is doing, although the extent of reporting may vary greatly.

In my own experience, those in managerial positions tend to prefer managerial supervision because they are more confident that it will be implemented. This experience is supported by Barker (1996), according to whom managers consider that the implementation of supervision must be organised in a top-down fashion, any other methods being regarded as logistically impossible. People in non-managerial positions, however, are often deeply suspicious of managers' motives and see supervision as a policing exercise. Even if those in management genuinely support the aims and objectives of supervision, regarding it as a way to support and help develop people, this may not be believed by their staff. This is probably due to the unique culture of nursing, which is usually not understood or appreciated by those outside it, although Shohet & Wilmot (1991) recognise that 'it is hard to have open supervision in a culture where there is a great deal of mistrust and talking behind backs' (p. 96).

My view is that if supervision in nursing is going to work, it must be consultative, a view which is often regarded as precious or over-idealistic by members of other professions such as counselling or social work. Brown & Bourne (1996), for example, in writing about supervision for social workers, take it as a given that supervision is managerial. They write:

> what distinguishes supervision from most other personal relationships is the formal authority and power vested in the supervisor by their role in the agency. It is a compulsory unequal relationship that has not been chosen by either person. It can also have a significant influence on the supervisee's future career. This power factor lies behind many of the distortions that can occur in the supervisory relationship, and which get in the way of effective productive work. (p. 82)

Despite its apparent acceptance by the social work profession, from the above quotation, it is clear that this type of managerial supervision is not without problems and limitations.

Regarding the counselling situation, Feltham & Dryden (1994) point out that where line management and supervision are identical, supervisors should realise that supervisees may not feel free to disclose personal material, and so the supervision is likely to be less effective than if it was offered by an outsider (p. 22). Jacobs (1996), discussing supervision in psychotherapy, reports that 'strenuous efforts are made in many settings to separate line management and supervision', making it possible for supervisees to talk about their work 'without any anxiety' (p.1). It would seem prudent, therefore, to learn from the experience of other professions and separate clinical supervision from managerial function. I agree with Kaberry (1992) who states that there is 'a distinction between line management and supervision', and that if this distinction is not clearly defined, 'nurses may fear that showing their mistakes, failures and negative feelings about patients would be detrimental to future promotion'. She goes on to say that if supervision is going to succeed in nursing, there will have to be changes in the underlying culture so that supervision is regarded as a valued part of the work (Kaberry 1992, van Ooijen 1994). In Chapter 5, I discuss how supervisors can handle potential problems between organisations and individual supervisees.

Choice of priority

Relevant to the type of supervision chosen is the question posed by Holloway (1995: 3) of which should be the priority: the organisation or the professional development of the supervisee? Although widespread, this type of dualistic 'either/or' thinking is not very helpful and is something we need to get away from. Before doing so, however, we need to understand the background to this type of thinking and the effect it has had on women in general and the nursing profession in particular.

Why do people engage in either/or thinking?

Dualistic thinking, which sees the world in terms of opposites, is inherent in our western world view and has its origins in the philosophy of Plato as well as the main religions of the western world, Christianity and Judaism. Somehow in the west it seems almost impossible to make sense of the world without resorting to opposites, such as black versus white, male versus female, good versus bad, rational versus emotional, and so on. Feminist writers have pointed out the effects this type of thinking has had on women who, because of their bodily functions associated with child bearing, came to be identified with the body and were therefore regarded as lacking rationality. Men, on the other hand, were seen as logical, rational and identified with the mind (Lloyd 1993). Lloyd and other feminist authors have discussed the undesirability of this state of affairs that has led to the world becoming predominantly male-oriented. Many women, and possibly men also, feel alienated as a large part of human experience is excluded from the rationalistic world view.

As far as health care is concerned, the dualistic thinking that characterises the rationalistic world view has contributed to the comparatively low status of nursing compared to that of medicine. This is because nursing is concerned with the body and with caring, whereas the goal of medicine is to cure. In other words, caring, which is seen as relying on non-rational emotion, sensitivity and being in touch with the body, is seen as clearly separate from and inferior to curing, which is regarded as a higher-order, scientific and rational activity. Although the nursing profession has made great strides in the past few decades, it is still at the receiving end of this dualistic distinction.

The effect on nursing

Nursing now appears to be in a 'twilight zone'. On the one hand it has traditionally been excluded from the public realm of management and the decision-making sphere, and on the other it has now also lost its place in the private sphere. Whereas in the past, matrons and ward sisters had control over the patients' environment, that control has now largely been lost and divided between domestic supervisors, catering managers and others. Actual nursing care itself is also being lost as the people in the public sphere of management are extending their power into the private realm of the patients. As a result, the number of qualified nurses is continuously decreasing, 'care' being delivered by less trained or untrained people. This development, which is due to the low value given to what nurses do, is in effect within the tradition of regarding the feminine and the particular as inferior to the male and the universal.

Implications for supervision

Within the current climate, the overriding principles of saving costs, improving patient throughput and achieving cure are paramount. It is my observation that nurses tend to perceive managers as downgrading the importance of patients' experience and need of care, in order to achieve these principles. Although the goals of supervision include the maintenance and enhancement of that care, in light of the above discussion it is important to be aware of the different positions from which nurses and managers view the concept.

Regarding the suspicion with which nurses often perceive managers' ideas for implementation, I feel it is imperative that both sides listen to each other and work out together the strategy most suited to their particular area. Top-down implementation may be viewed with suspicion, whereas bottom-up implementation may be problematic too, as the people concerned may be so occupied with doing the difficult task of day-to-day patient care that asking them to implement supervision would be perceived as 'yet another task to do'. Surprising it may seem, but it is not unusual for me to hear of ward managers who have been told that they have to implement supervision, without being given any funds, education or help. Although trusting people with such a task is encouraging, it is important that they are empowered to do so and given whatever means are needed.

Managerial supervision is often favoured by those charged with its implementation as it could be argued that supervision should be a part of the managerial role. This is not surprising since not very long ago, ward managers were regarded as having total responsibility for their area, which included all the staff. Consequently, managers kept a fairly tight reign on staff, were aware of their capabilities and shortcomings, and in effect did a great deal of checking up. In my view, the growing emphasis on the responsibility and autonomy of individual nurses themselves, coupled with the ever-increasing complexity, both technological and organisational, of health care delivery, has led to an erosion of the supervisory role of the ward manager. There has been some attempt to bring it back, by means of Individual Performance Review, for example, but this is at best only an annual exercise and therefore not a real substitute.

The erosion of the supervisory role of the ward manager has in some cases led to a decline in leadership, particularly as to be a ward manager came, in some cases, to be seen as just a step on the career ladder. In other words, in the past, to be a ward manager was the summit of what most nurses aimed for, and as a result many were very experienced. However, when it became a step on the career ladder, many ward managers were relatively young and inexperienced and therefore reluctant to undertake a strict supervisory role. Also, many people achieved leadership of a clinical area without any management training, or sometimes without any further education. Although this picture has changed in recent years, it is still possible that ward managers may have received less post-registration education than some of their staff, which can make managerial supervision problematic.

One result of the recent health care reforms has been a decline in the nursing career structure, meaning that, once again, many nurses may not move beyond the level of ward or unit manager. In my view, it is time that the crucial nature of that position is recognised and adequately rewarded. Also, in the present situation, it really is no longer good enough to expect people to function at a managerial level without receiving prior preparation. The given situation is too complex to continue to expect people to learn by trial and error; after all, we are dealing with people's lives and well-being.

Perhaps an ideal scenario would be to restore the ward manager's role to something most nurses would want to aim for and for which they would receive adequate preparation and renumeration. The role could include an element of supervision. However, this supervisory aspect of the managerial role would not be identical to professional supervision. As some of the authors quoted above have pointed out, managerial supervision goes only so far, and there is a limit to the extent to which people will be honest with the person who also does their individual performance review, and who can have a make-or-break effect on their career.

Ideally, therefore, I should like professional supervision to be totally separate from managerial supervision so that both can be as effective as possible. This does not mean that I wish to advocate an abandonment of the normative function of professional supervision; indeed an experienced nurse may well seek out a supervisor who is not afraid to perform this function. I see both supervisor and supervisee as having responsibility for the normative function, with supervisors enabling supervisees to look at their work afresh, by means of effective questioning and challenge.

Individual or group supervision

Apart from the choice between managerial or non-managerial supervision, there are other choices to be made, as supervision can be implemented in a number of different ways. Although organisations may prefer group supervision for efficiency reasons, I find that potential supervisees often express a preference for receiving personal supervision. It would seem useful to have both types of supervision available in an organisation as people's needs may vary. It is likely, for example, that once people have experienced one-to-one supervision for a number of years, they may feel sufficiently confident to try group supervision. Alternatively, some may prefer a combination of group and individual supervision. There really is no definitive blueprint; each person needs to decide what is likely to be most effective for him or her.

Advantages of individual supervision

1. confidentiality is less likely to be compromised
2. it may feel safer; people are likely to feel more comfortable
3. there is adequate time to really investigate an issue in detail

4. the relationship is likely to grow and develop over time, so as people get to know each and trust each other, they are likely to engage more honestly and at a deeper level.

Disadvantages of individual supervision

1. it is expensive in terms of time and resources
2. there is more opportunity for 'collusion', i.e. the supervisor may consciously or unwittingly fail to challenge the supervisee on areas where there is room for improvement
3. there is less likelihood of 'blind spots' being discovered
4. there is a danger of the supervisor 'riding hobbyhorses' (i.e., overfocusing on their favourite subjects at the expense of the supervisee's needs)
5. there is a possibility of becoming too cosy, or like a 'mutual appreciation society'
6. in cases of difficult issues the supervisor may feel pressurised, with no one to share the load.

Advantages of group supervision

1. It may be seen as a more economic use of time, money or expertise (but whether this view is correct is debatable).

2. It can be helpful to see that others have similar issues, problems or anxieties, which will make people feel less isolated.

3. Group members can learn from each other; also, supervisors can use the group to check out any parallel processes or intuitions. This is particularly useful for inexperienced supervisors who have not developed the confidence to trust their own perceptions.

4. A group may offer a wider range of professional as well as life experiences. It may also provide a good mix of age, gender, culture, race or personality types, which may be helpful in understanding issues and people brought for discussion and reflection.

5. A group is a good place to try out active techniques such as role play and sculpting. If a nurse wants to demonstrate a particular situation which involved more than two people, for example, members of the group may take on the roles of the people concerned. Equally, a group may be useful to try out different strategies or interventions, giving the supervisee honest feedback on his effectiveness. Alternatively, the supervisee may like to role play a patient or other person brought to supervision, in order to gain an understanding of that person's position, point of view and way of behaving.

Disadvantages of group supervision

1. However the group is structured, there will be less time for individual supervisees. Possibilities include dividing the time equally between those present, taking turns at being the supervisee for the session, agreeing a maximum number of people who can receive supervision in each session, and working this out democratically, or giving priority to those with the most urgent problem. Whereas all these are viable ways of managing group supervision, the individual will never have as much time, session by session, as with personal supervision. Without good facilitation of the group, there could be a danger of the less vocal or perhaps more ambivalent members of the group being overlooked and not receiving an equal share of supervision.

2. The second set of disadvantages concerns the dynamics of the group.

(a) The group may collude and prevent effective challenge.

(b) The group may resist deep reflection and jump in with premature advice as soon as an issue has been outlined.

(c) The group may wish to perpetuate the status quo and be a 'mutual admiration society' or, conversely, adopt an 'it's awful, but nothing can be done' attitude. These last two disadvantages are particularly likely if the facilitator is inexperienced in supervision, working with groups, or both.

(d) Conversely, the group may be competitive and challenging in a destructive manner.

(e) The group may become preoccupied with its own dynamics rather than with the supervisory process.

3. A group may be experienced as intimidating.

4. Revealing possible personal shortcomings to other nurses may seem almost inconceivable, as this is not traditionally part of the nursing culture. It may therefore be difficult to share anxieties or worries. It may well be that this is even more difficult for the more experienced nurses or those in more managerial positions.

5. In a group, people may worry more about confidentiality.

Clearly the way in which a group is supervised is crucial and supervisors need, therefore, to be experienced in the process of supervision and preferably also in handling groups. This is even more the case with peer group supervision, where members of the group take turns at being the supervisor. However, group members can help each other to develop these skills by giving honest feedback on how the group is facilitated. Thus a group can provide a useful learning experience, particularly when people decide to experiment with different techniques or try out different models of supervision. After all, as has been mentioned earlier, supervision can be play, and group supervision can provide a safe 'sandpit' in which to try out building different 'castles'. If they do not quite work, they are easily and painlessly knocked down and new ones put in their place. Also, the sandpit analogy aptly demonstrates the transience of any way of working. If supervision is going to remain dynamic, different ways of working are always useful and help keep people on their toes.

Team supervision

I should like to point out that group supervision is not the same as team supervision, which is in essence, managerial, if carried out by a line manager, although a team could also be facilitated by an outside facilitator. The advantages and disadvantages of group supervision apply equally to a team, but there are also a number of additional factors.

If the supervision is carried out by a manager, the disadvantages of managerial supervision apply equally and are possibly magnified. Also, as a team will by definition include people of different experience and grade who are related to each other in a hierarchy, people at both ends of the hierarchy may feel inhibited. The people in the lower positions may feel less inclined to discuss issues freely as they may fear it will affect how they are regarded professionally, which could damage their future job prospects. Conversely, people towards the top end of the scale may feel that they have a reputation to keep up and may find it difficult to share worries or anxieties with those for whom they have some managerial responsibility.

Also, if there are problems within a team it is likely that those dynamics will be played out in supervision, making it less effective. Although a skilled facilitator may be able to work with this by bringing it into the open, it is debatable whether supervision is really the appropriate forum for this. One solution may be to have team supervision in addition to individual supervision. This way the needs of individual team members are met, yet the team is also attended to. It may be a worthwhile idea to regard the team itself as an entity requiring supervision, as it is then up to the team and the manager/facilitator to decide what is or is not appropriate to include. If individual team members' supervisory needs are already catered for elsewhere, it may be good practice to include team building and team development in the contract. Clearly this type of supervision is quite demanding of the supervisor/facilitator and requires different skills than for individual or even group supervision. People certainly need to be experienced in handling groups and in managing any conflict that may rise to the surface. I stress the importance of adequate training here, as inadequate handling of groups or teams could have disastrous consequences and result in the exacerbation, rather than the resolution of problems and conflicts.

The importance of choice

In my view, it is not advisable to tell people that they should implement supervision without giving them any choice in the matter. An educational programme geared towards familiarising people with the concept of supervision should therefore be the first step. If supervision is going to work, it should not be experienced as imposed from above. Giving individual nurses a choice regarding the type of supervision as well as the person they would like as a supervisor is crucial. It is equally important that people are not coerced into being supervisors if they do not feel ready for this role, nor would it seem to be a good idea for potential supervisors to be told who they will be supervising. As can be seen in Chapter 6, where the process of supervision is discussed, one of the first tasks to be done by both supervisor and supervisee is to establish whether they can actually work together. Choosing by whom to be supervised also involves making a decision regarding the specialty or even the discipline of a supervisor.

There may be a link here with the developmental stage of the nurse as discussed in Chapter 1. If a nurse is still fairly inexperienced or perhaps new to a specialty, it may be advisable to receive supervision from someone who is familiar with that specialty. As experience and confidence are gained, however, it can often be more useful to seek supervision from someone whose experience is completely different. If a nurse who works in intensive care, for example, is supervised by a nurse who works in a GP practice, it will be necessary for the supervisor to ask all kinds of questions in order to get to grips with the work situation of the supervisee. Whereas this may seem at first sight a waste of time, this is not actually the case as, paradoxically, the very fact that the supervisor may ask some seemingly naive questions enables the supervisee to see the situation afresh. I have found time and again that supervisors from different specialties are often more effective in challenging people's work practices, thus illuminating blind spots, whereas supervisors from the same specialty may share those blind spots and may be just as stuck on the same issue.

Some people may decide to go even further and seek supervision from someone who is not a nurse. A fairly senior nurse, for example, may feel that it is useful to seek supervision from a (non-line) manager as long as that person is familiar with the concept of professional supervision and has the necessary skills. People whose roles include a substantial psychological element, such as community psychiatric nurses, or nurses working in rehabilitation or palliative care, may benefit from supervision by someone from a related discipline such as a clinical psychologist, psychiatrist or psychotherapist. Conversely, in theory, there is no reason why an experienced nurse with good supervisory skills should not supervise someone from another discipline if that seems useful and acceptable to both.

More important than the clinical area, specialty or even discipline of the supervisor is her ability to supervise. In other words, she needs to understand what supervision is about and have the necessary experience and skills to be effective. The supervisor also needs to be working according to a model, whether it is a recognised model such as those discussed in Chapter 1, or one that she has developed herself by integrating those models that she finds helpful. I stress the importance of a model as without some kind of framework the supervision could easily lose its way and fail to be effective.

POWER

Except perhaps in peer supervision, it is my belief that the concept of power is intrinsic to the supervisory relationship. Even in consultative supervisory relationships where a fee is paid, it is difficult to escape the issue of power. This may be an unpalatable truth for many people, but to deny it merely causes the issue to go underground, from where it can then sabotage the effectiveness of the process. The most successful supervisory relationships are those where any possible inequality or power relations are acknowledged, while at the same time every effort is made to minimise their effect in practice.

In addition to the supervisory relationship itself involving an imbalance of power, there are other relevant factors such as age, gender, sexual orientation, race, class, cultural background, education and managerial or occupational position. Although nursing is a largely female occupation, it will come as no surprise to anyone to learn that the higher up in the hierarchy one goes, the more men will be encountered. Although feminism has had an effect on the status of women, our western world is still by and large a male-dominated world, in which women have to work very hard to achieve status and credibility. As a consequence, many women do not feel as confident about themselves as they should, underestimate their achievements and often have low self-esteem. Nurses are no different, and the low status of nursing and the lack of influence the profession seems to have on the health service as a whole only serve as reminders that women still have a long way to go before they are regarded as truly equal to men.

Therefore, if a man supervises a woman, the power imbalance is intensified, unless the supervisor consciously attempts to equalise the situation. A woman supervising a man may find herself behaving differently than she does with female supervisees. She may find it more difficult to challenge a man, or conversely, may overcompensate and become overly critical or demanding. In addition, each person comes with his or his own history of relationships with the opposite sex, which may help or hinder the supervision process.

The following scenario is an example of what might happen.

Mark, a mature, newly qualified psychiatric nurse, had chosen Eleanor, a clinical psychologist, as his supervisor. As he had already gained a degree in psychology before entering nurse education, Mark felt that Eleanor was an appropriate person, from whom he could learn a great deal. Eleanor, on her part, was pleased to supervise Mark, as he was obviously very bright and capable and had already established an excellent reputation. They contracted for six sessions of one and a half hours a month, after which they would have a review in order to see whether their way of working was effective and satisfactory for both.

On the evaluation day, both were nervous and initially reluctant to be honest. However, after having praised each other for a while, Eleanor said 'Mark, we are both obviously pleased with the way things have been going, but I am aware of feeling somewhat uncomfortable with this. I have a feeling that there is something we are not addressing. Does this ring any bells with you?'

Mark thought for a moment and then said, 'Well, yes, actually but I am not quite sure how to say it. OK, here goes. Before I met you I was very in awe of you as I had been told you were this very intelligent and powerful women, so I must have been a bit of a masochist as powerful women really scare me. However, I felt you were the best person for the job so I went for it anyway. On meeting you though, I found you very approachable and not all the ogre some people led me to believe you were. You have been very supportive, and I have already learnt a great deal. I like the way you let me come to my own conclusions, only coming in with advice when I am stuck. So what I am going to say will feel strange. What I would like is more challenge, I feel that you are almost too nice to me and I could cope with a more robust approach. I am not asking for criticism, but I suppose I am asking to be stretched a little more.'

Eleanor was surprised, she had no idea that Mark had been in awe of her as he always seemed so confident. In fact, his very confidence, and the fact that he had a degree in psychology and had taught the subject for a few years, had made her feel quite nervous about supervising him. He was also a few years older than her, which contributed to her lack of confidence. She had compensated for this by pretending to be very confident and knowledgeable, but in truth she was afraid to challenge Mark properly. Also she was afraid of being found to be wrong, which was why she tried to get Mark to solve his own issues. Whereas the latter certainly was in Mark's case the right approach, the lack of challenge did mean that on occasion she had let things slip by that she should have brought to his attention.

However, having discussed the relationship and the way they were working openly, both Mark and Eleanor now felt much clearer about each other's position. In fact, they contracted to build in evaluation of the process itself as ongoing rather than only once in a while, both parties being at liberty to comment on how the process was going whenever they felt it to be appropriate.

In addition to gender, racial or cultural background is also an important issue to acknowledge, although research into the effects of mixed race/culture supervision is very limited (Leong & Wagner 1994). Many people these days pretend to be 'colour-blind' and would say that a person's colour, race or culture does not make a difference. This is laudable but not entirely honest. We all form impressions of people depending on their appearance and background, since particularly when we first meet them, that is all we have to go on. Brown & Bourne (1996) advocate an 'anti-oppressive approach' to supervision, with the supervisor communicating a 'fundamental belief in the potential and ability of each supervisee' (p. 37). This does not mean, however, that the supervisor will collude with the supervisee if his work is not all it should be, as this would clearly be disadvantageous.

Sometimes people are nervous of challenging those from other cultures for fear of being accused of racism or discrimination. However, in addition to support, supervision is also about the safeguarding of professional standards, which will mean at times confronting a supervisee if these standards are not being met. It is important to remember that confrontation should be done constructively rather than destructively. A skilled supervisor will not be afraid to confront a supervisee with a difficult issue, but will at the same time show that she values him as a person, and gives recognition to any other contributory factors such as organisational problems (Brown & Bourne 1996). Honesty is crucial. If people know that the supervisor is genuine, does not have an axe to grind and can be trusted to do whatever is appropriate, be it support, praise, challenge or confront, then they are much more likely to accept constructive criticism.

What I am really talking about here is maturity. Not being afraid to challenge or confront when necessary is really saying to the supervisee 'I value you as a mature human being who can cope with the truth and who will react appropriately'. Conversely, being afraid to challenge is giving the opposite message. In other words, if supervisors are afraid to challenge anyone from a different gender, class, colour or cultural background, they are in effect saying 'I do not think you are mature enough to cope with honest feedback, so I will treat you with kid gloves just in case you fall apart'. So an anti-discriminatory approach means valuing each person as a mature individual and not treating people from other backgrounds as somehow less mature or inferior. Cook & Helms (1988), in a study of

225 supervisees from different ethnic backgrounds, found that irrespective of the cultural background of either supervisor or supervisee, feeling liked by the supervisor was an important determinant of satisfaction. As part of the preparation to become a supervisor, it would therefore be useful to foster the development of cross-cultural awareness and the impact that race and culture can have on people's working lives, as well as their lives in general.

An anti-discriminatory way of working is in line with the humanist ideal underlying nursing in that it values each person as a unique individual, whatever his or her background (Rogers 1951; Burnard 1985). Recently, however, the humanist philosophy has been attacked by Mulholland (1995) as having the potential of leading to a culture of extreme individualism or even victimisation, as the individual is seen as ultimately responsible for his or her predicament. Mulholland further argues that nursing models that are based on humanist principles have downplayed the effects of race and culture, and their relationship to power. The extreme form of humanism as outlined by Mulholland is obviously to be avoided and, is in any case, a result of misunderstanding its philosophy. There is, however, some truth in his view of nursing having closed its eyes to the subject of race and culture and the need for an awareness of issues of power. What is needed, therefore, is an open debate on all aspects of power and discrimination, not only between each supervisee and supervisor, but also within the nursing profession as a whole. If relevant factors are acknowledged, and any resulting inequalities are 'put on the table', as it were, and openly debated, they will 'lose their power'. In other words, there has to be a constant striving for equality.

Who owns the session?

Related to power is the issue of who owns the supervision session. In other words, who has the responsibility for the session regarding what is discussed, timing, boundaries, and so on? If a relationship is truly equal, it would seem that supervisor and supervisee share the responsibility. However, this is only possible in consulative supervision; it is difficult to see how one could have a truly equal relationship if one's supervisor is also one's manager. Also, for supervisees new to the process, it may be unfair to expect them to take equal responsibility as they lack the experience of what is involved. However, the aim here should be to regard the process as developmental, with the supervisee taking increasing responsibility as he gains experience. Supervisors need therefore to be flexible and to be aware of each supervisee's capability and developmental stage. Issues of responsibility may usefully be included in the contract (see p. 47).

DEVELOPMENT OF THE RELATIONSHIP

How to start: beginning phase

If the supervisory relationship is going to work, adequate preparation is essential. First of all, the supervisee needs to be clear about what it is he wants and needs from supervision. Then he needs to look around for the kind of person who is likely to be able to meet these needs. It is good practice to shop around before embarking on supervision in order to ensure that the process will be as useful as possible. In other words, in order to find out what kind of people are available and what they have to offer, it is necessary to meet them and have exploratory conversations. Within the counselling and psychotherapy professions this is normal practice, and a first meeting is always regarded as exploratory, with both parties asking themselves the question 'what would it be like to work with this person?

As regular supervision involves a considerable commitment in terms of time as well as personal involvement, feeling good about each other is essential. During an exploratory meeting, both parties need to be honest about their experience, expertise, style of working and preferred ways of relating. Some people, for example, may like to be challenged, whereas others prefer a more supportive approach. Views on nursing need also to be discussed; while it is not necessary for both parties to come from the same specialty, it is important that they see eye to eye regarding what nursing is and is about. If a supervisor believes, for example, that nurses should never become involved in patients' emotional needs as that would prevent them from giving good physical and technical care, they are unlikely to be helpful to a supervisee whose specialty is supporting people through the experience of cancer, for example.

Whereas this example may seem rather extreme, it is important that both parties know what they are talking about when they discuss how they work with people. So an introductory meeting must not be rushed and may easily take an hour. If, after meeting, say, three potential supervisors, the supervisee feels more drawn to one of them, another meeting needs to take place to discuss a contract – assuming, of course, that the supervisor also feels that she can work with this particular supervisee.

Contracting

Before starting out on supervision, it is important to discuss the aims, goals and expectations of both parties, as failure to do this may lead to one or both ending up dissatisfied (Barker 1996). The contract needs to be fairly detailed so that both parties know exactly where they stand. When things go wrong in supervision, it is often due to the contract not being sufficiently clear so that misunderstandings arise. It is useful to subdivide a contract into a few main areas:

- logistics or ground rules
- limits and boundaries
- accountability
- aims and goals
- responsibilities
- preferred process.

Logistics or ground rules

These include first of all logistics of time and place. Deciding how often to meet, for how long and where seems fairly obvious. What tends to get overlooked is how to handle cancellation or postponement of meetings, although a note of caution is appropriate here. There needs to be commitment to supervision; if this is absent there is a real danger that supervision will be sacrificed when other work matters seem more urgent or pressing. Supervisors who work privately often have a minimum notice time, which means that if the supervisee cancels the meeting within a certain period, such as 24 or even 48 hours, the agreed fee must still be paid. It is easy to understand why this should be the case as supervisors in this position depend on the people they see for their income. If a session gets cancelled without adequate notice, that time cannot be filled and there is loss of income.

However, similar considerations are relevant when supervisor and supervisee work for the same organisation. Although no actual money changes hands, there is an issue of time planning and organisation. If a supervisor has freed up time to spend an hour on supervision, and then receives a cancellation five minutes prior to the meeting, it may not be possible to use that hour effectively. With adequate notice, however, the supervisor will be able to rearrange the time so that there is no loss either to her or to the organisation. Naturally, the argument applies equally to supervisees.

Limits and boundaries

Confidentiality. Confidentiality is an absolutely crucial factor to discuss. It is not sufficient to simply say or assume that the sessions will be totally confidential, as that is never true. Nurses supervising nurses will be bound by the UKCC Code of Conduct which clearly stipulates the limits to confidentiality (United Kingdom Central Council for Nursing, Midwifery and Health Visiting 1992). However, the Code discusses issues only in general and there is room for individual interpretation. Ultimately it is up to each and every professional nurse how he interprets a situation in light of the Code. This needs to be discussed before embarking on supervision. Both supervisor and supervisee need to agree a procedure for possible breaches of the Code and discuss who has responsibility for what.

A useful way of working would be for the supervisor to make it clear that in cases of breaches of the Code she would be unable to collude with pretending it had not happened. However, rather than taking the situation out of the hands of the supervisee, which would clearly be disempowering, she would help the supervisee to take the action she considers to be appropriate in the situation. Only in a case where the supervisee would be unwilling to do this might a supervisor take action herself. If these factors are discussed in detail beforehand, it is then up to the supervisee whether he decides to discuss certain issues with the supervisor.

Another way of working would be for the supervisor to state that she does not want to hear about breaches of the Code, in other words, issues involving a breach of the Code of Conduct would fall outside the boundaries of supervision. This in fact sometimes happens with group supervision if one or more group members feel that they do not want to be placed in a situation where, having heard about an issue, they may have to take action. Supervisors who are not nurses are not bound by the Code of Conduct, but may have a professional code of their own as well as an obligation to abide by the law of the land.

In my experience, some people are dismayed and may react angrily when they find out that there are limits to the confidentiality that is possible within supervision, and they may insist that the supervision will not work. Although understandable, this is an overreaction which is not borne out by facts. Most nurses are conscientious people who uphold the Code of Conduct. However, it is perhaps not surprising that they feel uncomfortable with taking action where they have observed unprofessional practice, as they do not wish to cause trouble for a colleague. In supervision, they can be helped to see that once they are aware of a problem, they are actually implicated themselves unless they take action. Thus, even in cases where confidentiality may need to be broken, it is clear that the aim of supervision is to safeguard good practice. Conversely, having regular supervision will help nurses to examine their practice and become more conscious of what they are doing, which will help to prevent breaches of the Code.

Although it may be true, as has sometimes been stated, that no amount of supervision would have prevented tragedies such as those in the case of Beverly Allitt*, it is equally possible that a skilled supervisor would have picked up that something was amiss from the way practice was talked about. What the Allitt case also clearly demonstrates is the need for good management as well as clinical supervision.

Beverly Allitt was an enrolled nurse who was convicted of murdering four babies, attempting to murder three more, and causing grievous bodily harm to six. Her actions, which took place over a period of two months, involved wrongly injecting the children with insulin. A subsequent government enquiry criticised staffing levels as well as the lack of leadership and poor management. As a result of the enquiry thirteen recommendations were made which included careful pre-employment screening. Within the nursing press, however, it was suggested that this would be insufficient and that more needed to be done in terms of monitoring of practice and effective clinical supervision (Naish 1997).

Note taking is another issue to be discussed. Some people are unhappy about any notes being taken, feeling that this is likely to compromise confidentiality. Others, particularly if they supervise more than one person, may feel it necessary to keep notes not only as an aide memoire, but also as a means for reflection on how they are performing as supervisors. Sometimes both parties show each other their notes at regular intervals; others do not feel this need. What needs to be discussed is the purpose of keeping notes, as both parties need to be clear what the notes are needed for. If a supervisee, for example, is unhappy with the idea of notes being kept, then the supervisor should agree not to do so. However, the supervisee may then on occasion find that the supervisor does not necessarily recall all that has been discussed, and may need a certain amount of prompting.

Keeping notes can be very useful for evaluation purposes. If evaluation is carried out regularly, say every six sessions, notes are very helpful. It is surprising how easy it is to forget issues once they have been resolved. Also, the supervisee may find that keeping notes or a reflective diary helps with compiling his Professional Portfolio as well as with preparation for Individual Performance Review, as successes and achievements are being recorded.

Storage may be an issue. Clearly, no one except the individuals concerned should have access to any notes or diaries, so unless one has the use of a locked cabinet (as well as the only key), it may be prudent not to keep these files in one's work area.

Other boundaries. The desired balance between the three functions of supervision also needs to be discussed during contracting. Although supervision is meant to be supportive, with the supervisor endeavouring to listen attentively and accurately with empathy and understanding, it would be inappropriate for this to lead the supervisor to 'therapise' the nurse. It is therefore important to realise the difference between counselling, therapy and supervision and to establish where one ends and the other begins. The difference between supervision and counselling is a commonly debated issue which indicates that within nursing there is a certain amount of confusion about the nature of counselling.

Although individual supervisory pairs need to decide between them what they feel is appropriate to supervision and what is not, it is possible to draw a clear boundary. Supervision is concerned with nursing; counselling with the person. In other words, the focus, indeed the purpose of supervision is to help the nurse reflect on practice in order to both maintain and improve professional standards. Whereas being helped to reflect in this way is supportive, it is not the same as counselling.

In counselling, people are helped to 'help themselves' with issues that bother them, such as grief, relationship and or sexual problems, having been abused or being depressed without specifically knowing why. Counselling involves being with people while they look inside themselves and find out what they are really feeling or experiencing. So in counselling, the focus is the person, whereas in supervision it is the work. It would be inappropriate, indeed dangerous for a supervisor to start delving into a nurse's personal history of, say, sexual abuse. First of all, the situation would be very likely to get out of hand, but secondly, the supervisee might well feel very embarrassed afterwards and not wish to continue being supervised by the same person. Indeed, 'being therapised' is what potential supervisees most often fear about supervision.

The British Association for Counselling (BAC) has recognised the importance of keeping the two activities separate, and has ruled that no one should act as counsellor and supervisor to the same person, as it would be impossible to prevent boundaries from blurring (BAC 1996).

Some of the confusion may be due to the fact that although there are clear distinctions between supervision and counselling, both activities involve listening. Good listening skills (also sometimes called basic counselling skills) are essential both to counselling and supervision. Indeed, it could be argued that every nurse really ought to have these skills. However, using listening or basic counselling skills is not the same as counselling. This would be the same as saying that being able to perform some 'basic nursing care', such as bathing a patient, performing some mouth care and making beds, is the same as nursing. They are essential skills, but are only a very small part of the whole picture.

In order to maintain supervision as a professional alliance between equals, it is advisable to agree shared responsibility for the maintenance of boundaries. If this is not done and the supervisee hands over responsibility to the supervisor there is the potential for the misuse of power, however unintentional this may be.

Accountability

Who is accountable for what and to whom must also be part of the contract. Although, as has been pointed out, all nurses are bound to practise within the UKCC Code of Conduct, more local issues of accountability may very depending on agreements with and expectations of the employer. Some employers may request that supervisors report on the progress of supervisees or on their perceived level of practice. This may be appropriate where supervision is part of education, or where the supervisor also has a managerial role. However, in other cases it is advisable for supervisors to think very carefully before agreeing to such requests, as this is likely to seriously affect the nature of the relationship and the effectiveness of the supervision. It is therefore essential that who is accountable for what is made clear in the contract discussions. Generally, supervisees are accountable for their own practice. However, it may be useful to discuss what procedure to follow should any action ever need to be taken by the supervisor. If these issues are talked about frankly prior to commencing supervision, it will make things much easier should a difficult situation arise.

Aims and goals

As discussed earlier, both parties need to be clear about how they see the purpose of supervision. In other words, what is supervision for, and what can be achieved, both in individual sessions and in the long term? This needs to be discussed, including agreement on the desired balance between the three functions of supervision – support, education and development – and the maintenance and enhancement of the work.

Responsibilities

It is important to be clear on who sets the agenda: is it the supervisor or the supervisee? Some supervisors like to develop a long-term plan with supervisees regarding the kind of issues and aspects of the job to be looked at. This often involves knowing beforehand what is going to be discussed in a particular session. Others are happy to work with whatever the supervisee brings on the day, feeling that as supervision is for the benefit of the supervisee, he should be the one to decide what it is he needs.

Both views have merit and it is up to the people concerned to decide between them how they are going to work.

Preferred process

This will include some of the elements discussed above such as the balance between support and challenge, as well as the three functions of supervision. It also involves deciding whether to work to a particular model or structure, and if so, which one. Sometimes pairs new to supervision decide to contract for trying out different methods. For example, people may decide to run six sessions according to Johns' model of reflection and then evaluate the advantages and disadvantages of working according to this method (Johns, 1997). For the next six sessions, they may then try out another model, and so on. It may also be useful to discuss what tools and methods both feel to be appropriate. Some people may only be comfortable with discussions, whereas others may wish to use experiential methods such as role play, art work, or other creative techniques.

How and when to evaluate also need to be included in the contract. It is good practice, particularly when still learning how to supervise but also as a general way of working, to evaluate each session briefly. What worked, what did not work, which interventions were really useful, which ones did not go anywhere, and so on. Both parties should be clear with each other and give honest feedback. If a supervisor feels that a supervisee was not really engaging in a session, expecting the supervisor to do all the work, this should be made clear. Conversely, a supervisee may feel that the supervisor is not sufficiently engaged, does not listen properly or is too quick to offer solutions. It is important to give each other this kind of feedback as without it, the supervision will not be as effective as it can be. In addition to sessional evaluation it is also useful to evaluate on a more long-term basis, say, every six sessions. 'How have we been working?', 'How is the relationship developing?', 'Is there anything we need to renegotiate?', are pertinent topics to discuss in such evaluations. Being clear on what is happening in the process of supervision as well as how it is developing is helpful, not only for the people concerned but also for the organisation. It would not seem unreasonable for an organisation to ask people involved in supervision: 'Tell us about three benefits that you can identify from having received supervision'.

ISSUES, LEARNING OPPORTUNITIES AND PROBLEMS

In this section, some potential problems or areas of difficulty that may occur in supervision are discussed. As I have pointed out earlier, we do not have to try to be perfect on every occasion as this would result in unnecessary pressure. What is important, however, is that we remain open to looking at ourselves and our performance with the willingness to learn from whatever happens. Thus every potential problem or sticking point becomes a learning opportunity, in fact, something positive rather than something to beat ourselves over the head about.

The supervisor who disempowers

Some supervisors disempower their supervisees through sheer enthusiasm. They are so keen do be seen to be doing a good job that they are over-eager and do not give supervisees sufficient space to find their own solutions. This is very common, especially with novice supervisors, and is probably due to the way in which nurses are prepared during their training. After all, nursing is sometimes described as a 'problem-solving activity', implying that if there is a problem, we as nurses have to solve it. Leaving aside the issue of whether that is the way things should be with patients, in supervision this approach is not helpful, or at least not if the supervisor is doing it all.

Related to being over-eager is the supervisor who needs to shine or show off, for whatever reasons. Perhaps she cannot wait to let people have the benefit of her insight, knowledge and experience. Another reason for the need to shine or show off is perhaps a feeling of insecurity, particularly as the supervisory role will be fairly new to most nurses.

Over-eager supervisors may also have a tendency to over-interpret, to feel that they can see the situation more clearly than the supervisee and understand all the intricacies and ramifications. It is certainly true that when we are in the middle of a situation it can be difficult to see the wood for the trees, and that the way out is to stand back and take a more objective point of view. However, this does not necessarily mean that an outsider has a clearer view: ultimately it is the supervisee who brings the issue and who is likely to have the most knowledge, however confused he may appear to be at first. Even if a supervisor is clear and does see things correctly, it is important to help the supervisee to develop the insight himself in order not to disempower him, and be sure that he really understands the situation and is not simply accepting what someone else is saying.

Keeping supervisees in a 'learner mode' is another trap that can befall very keen supervisors, especially if the supervisor is very experienced and loves imparting her knowledge. However, as was seen in Chapter 1, there is a developmental angle to supervision, with the relationship becoming more equal as the supervisee gains more experience.

The following scenario is an example of what can happen with some of the pitfalls outlined above.

Annie, a community psychiatric nurse, was telling her supervisor Hugh about how she was working with one of her clients. Although Annie was normally easy-going, perhaps somewhat dependent, she suddenly became interested in the issue of control when Hugh said: 'So he appears to be taking control of how you are working together'. Normally Annie would have said something like: 'Yes, I suppose so, is that all right?' or 'Oh, I had not looked at it like that' and leave it at that. This time, however, she said: 'What exactly is it with control? What is it? Should I be in control? Some people have told me that they feel the nurse should always be in control of any situation. We had a discussion about this in work recently and one of my managers was branded as a "control freak". At the same time two of my colleagues who are doing a counselling course say that they have been taught the "non-directive approach" which apparently means that control is in the hands of the patient. I feel very confused, I have always felt that I need to be in control and have felt lost when I have not been able to'.

All this happened towards the end of the contracted time. Hugh felt surprised and somewhat irritated. There were only 10 minutes left, and he felt that they had not yet completed the reflection and he was afraid that the session would overrun. Normally, Hugh was very clear on boundaries and always ended sessions on time. On this occasion, however, they ended up spending 15 minutes longer than usual and Hugh only managed to end the session by telling Annie that he was running late for another appointment.

As an experienced supervisor, Hugh had quite a few supervisees and had therefore arranged for specific supervision for his own supervision practice (as well as for his practice in general).

At his next session with Marge, his supervisor, he discussed what had happened with Annie and how baffled he was by her unusual behaviour as well as his own in letting the session overrun.

Hugh: 'I don't understand what happened with Annie last time.'

Marge: 'You look confused, what happened?'

Hugh: 'Well, as you know she's normally so quiet that I have been quite frustrated. After we talked about her last time I have worked hard to "bring her out" and get her to come up with ideas, but it has been hard going.'

Marge: 'Say a bit more?'

Hugh: 'Well, I like to think that I'm non-threatening and I always am at pains to give positive strokes, where they are deserved and where people's confidence needs boosting. Normally this works well and as people get used to me they grow in confidence and take a very active part in the process. But with Annie, there appears to have been very little development. She still has hardly any ideas of her own and seems to look to me for ideas and answers to her problems with clients. I don't like working in this way as I am a strong believer in helping people to find their own solutions and ways of working, but with Annie I somehow always seem to end up telling her what to do and teaching her things that I am often surprised she does not seem to know.'

Marge: 'Aha.'

Hugh: 'What do you mean, aha?'

Marge: 'Well, I was just wondering who is actually in control here?'

Hugh: 'Who is in control? Well me ... ah ... I see what you mean. Mmmmmm, I will have to think about this. Suddenly I feel quite manipulated.'

Marge: 'I wonder how Annie feels?'

Hugh: 'What do you mean?'

Marge: 'Well, you seem to feel that she has been controlling you, and certainly she appeared to do so in that last session, but I wonder how she feels normally. Perhaps we could role play this ... let's see, if you are Annie and I am you ... let's see where that will lead.'

During the ensuing role play, Hugh (as Annie) realised that he was quite intimidating as a supervisor and that in the last session Annie, probably quite unconsciously, told him that she wanted more control and would take it by stealth if it was not freely given. He determined to address the relationship during the next session and to investigate what in his behaviour caused her to feel intimidated and controlled.

Lack of commitment

This can be a major reason for supervision not being effective. If contracting has been carried out effectively and both parties are clear on what to expect from one another, commitment is more likely than if the contracting has been half-hearted. When problems of logistics do occur it is often useful to look back at the original contract to see if both are as clear as they should be.

If boundaries of time have not been agreed sufficiently, for example, people may come late (or even early), expecting the other person to accommodate this. Clearly this is not satisfactory as not only is waiting around for people to turn up not an effective use of time, it is also likely to make people feel annoyed and not in a mood to be helpful and supportive. Cancellation is another problem. If supervision is going to work, the time set aside should be protected and not sacrificed as soon as another urgent matter occurs. However, this may be difficult if colleagues are not in favour of supervision (Butterworth et al 1997).

Reasons for lack of commitment may lie in the method of implementation. If supervision is seen as a managerial control exercise or if the people involved have not had sufficient choice, they may react by passive resistance and by giving priority to other matters. Lack of commitment does not only show up in coming late or cancelling sessions, it can also manifest itself through insufficient engagement in the session itself, or merely paying lip service. However, if every session is evaluated and both parties give each other honest feedback, such issues will soon be out in the open and can therefore be dealt with as appropriate. If someone really does not want supervision and cannot be persuaded to give it an honest try, then it would seem that there is little point in continuing. However, this does not happen often. If people are honest with each other and are prepared to learn from feedback and mistakes, it seems that even the most skeptical people are eventually won over.

Supervisees who want to 'hide'

Sometimes supervisees may not feel comfortable talking about their practice, perhaps because they do not feel confident and are afraid to be criticised. They may be reluctant to engage in any meaningful reflection, saying that everything is 'fine' and there are 'no problems'. In fact, seeing supervision as a problem-solving exercise may also mean that a lack of problems at the time of supervision may lead to cancellation of the session. It is crucial therefore that at the start of supervision, both parties discuss their views of supervision and appreciate that it is to reflect on all aspects of practice, whether good or not so good.

Other people may want to hide because they are perfectionists and find it hard to admit to not always coming up to the mark. Women particularly tend to feel that they have to be perfect in every way, and if they are not, their self-esteem plummets. For such people, supportive supervision is extremely helpful. The need to be perfect all the time is a particularly heavy burden to carry and likely to eventually lead to burnout. Being given permission to not be perfect all the time, but to be 'good enough' can be wonderfully liberating and a great stress reliever.

Lastly, some supervisees may want to 'hide' because they feel threatened by the supervisor. If the supervisor is also their manager, for example, they may feel unhappy to disclose any shortcomings because of possible repercussions. Another reason may be low self-esteem or feelings of inadequacy on the part of the supervisee, leading to any questions or queries being seen as critical, even when they are not meant as such. Again, giving each other honest feedback may be helpful here. Supervisors can help by being very sensitive to how supervisees are feeling and helping them to see the positives in what they do. Being given recognition for what is done well will help develop people's feelings of self-worth and will also help them to look at areas that may need development.

CONCLUSION

The supervisory relationship is about being honest, mature, aware and safe. Any relationship is continuously being recreated in every moment and is likely to change and develop as time goes on. Regular evaluation is important to ensure that the process stays new, fresh and effective, and to avoid both parties getting into a rut or becoming complacent. It is, however, a good idea to change supervisor from time to time, say every two or three years. This is because no matter how well it is working, a certain amount of familiarity will develop. Changing regularly will keep the process alive. It is also a good method of learning as people have alternative ways of working and different things to offer. Finally, it should be clear that supervision involves a great deal of knowledge and experience and that careful preparation is therefore essential. Chapters 3 and 4 are therefore devoted to how we can prepare ourselves to take on the role of either supervisor or supervisee.

REFERENCES

British Association for Counselling 1996 Code of ethics and practice for supervisors of counsellors. BAC, Rugby

Barker P 1996 An overview of clinical supervision. Paper presented to the conference 'Clinical Supervision' presented by South East Wales Institute of Nursing and Midwifery Education, University of Wales College of Medicine and Cardiff Community Health Care Trust, 22 May, Cardiff

Brown A, Bourne I 1996 The social work supervisor. Open University Press, Buckingham

Burnard P 1985 Learning human skills: a guide for nurses. Heinemann, London

Butterworth T, Carson J, White E, Jeacock J, Clements A, Bishop V 1997 It is good to talk. An evaluation study in England and Scotland. Clinical supervision and mentorship. School of Nursing, Midwifery and Health Visiting, University of Manchester

Carroll M 1996 Counselling supervision, theory, skills and practice. Cassell, London

Clothier C, MacDonald C A, Shaw D A 1994 The Allitt inquiry. Her Majesty's Stationary Office (HMSO), London, p. 128–130

Cook D A, Helms J E 1988 Visible racial/ethnic group supervisees' satisfaction with cross-cultural supervision as predicted by relationship characteristics. Journal of Counselling Psychology 35(3): 268–274

Feltham C, Dryden W 1994 Developing counselling supervision. Sage, London

Jacobs M (ed) 1996 In search of supervision. Open University Press, Buckingham

Johns C 1997 Reflective practice and clinical supervision. Part 1: The reflective turn. European Nurse 2(2): 87–97

Kaberry S 1992 Supervision – support for nurses? Senior Nurse 12(5): 38–40

Leong F T L, Wagner N S 1994 Cross-cultural counselling supervision: what do we know? What do we need to know? Counselor Education and Supervision. 34 (December): 117–131

Lloyd G 1993 The man of reason, 'male' and 'female' in western philosophy. Routledge, London

Mulholland J 1995 Nursing, humanism and transcultural theory: the 'bracketing-out' of reality. Journal of Advanced Nursing 22: 442–449

Naish J 1997 Dangerous assumptions. Nursing Times 93(46): 37–38

Rogers C 1951 Client centred therapy. Constable, London
Shohet R, Wilmot J 1991 The key issue in the supervision of counsellors: the
    supervisory relationship. In: Dryden W, Thorne B (eds) Training and
    supervision for counselling in action. Sage, London
United Kingdom Council for Nursing, Midwifery and Health Visiting 1992 Code
    of conduct for the nurse, midwife and health Visitor. UKCC, London
van Ooijen E G 1994 Whipping up a storm. Nursing Standard 9(8): 48

3

Becoming a supervisee

How to prepare yourself to get the most out of supervision.

A great deal has been written on the concept of supervision, how to implement it and how to become a supervisor. In contrast, there does not appear to be much literature that focuses on the role of supervisees, how people can best prepare themselves for the role, what supervision is about and what it is reasonable to expect. Somehow, there appears to be a tacit assumption that the supervisor does all the work and all the supervisee has to do is to turn up for sessions. Such a passive view of supervision is not only erroneous, it is also unhelpful and not in tune with the role of the modern nurse as an autonomous professional. Being a supervisee is hard work, but it is also extremely rewarding. And, as with most things, the more people are prepared to put into it, the more they will get out of it.

Training for supervision should therefore not only be geared towards the skills and knowledge needed to become a supervisor, but also include what is needed to be an effective supervisee. Indeed, if possible, it would be preferable if people received supervision themselves before undertaking the role of supervisor, as much can be learnt from being at the receiving end of supervision. Eventually it is hoped that most nurses will have supervision for their work, with a substantial number also providing supervision for others.

In this chapter, I discuss the need for self-awareness, then there is a discussion on how to identify supervisory needs, followed by a description of more specific preparation needed to get maximum benefit from supervision.

In order to be directly useful, this chapter, as well as the next chapter on becoming a supervisor is written in a participative rather than an academic style and contains a number of activities. The reader may choose to first read through the entire chapter before carrying out the activities, or stop and complete each activity before going on. Keeping a reflective diary is recognised as an effective method of enhancing the ability to reflect (Boud et al 1985, Richardson & Maltby 1995), and I suggest that you keep a reflective diary while working through these chapters, in which to record the activities and any thoughts on the material presented.

SELF-AWARENESS: THE NEED FOR SUPPORT

Nursing may be described as a therapy in its own right. Indeed, the way in which nurses work and how they are with patients is thought to influence the patients' well-being. The term 'being with' or 'presencing' has been coined by several authors (Halldorsdottir 1991) and a number of prominent nurse theorists see how we 'are' with people as fundamental to caring (Watson 1985, Benner & Wrubel 1989).

This is a far cry from the hopefully outdated view of 'professional' nursing as described in the now classic study by Menzies Lyth (1988), according to which, it was important to keep a professional distance. Of course keeping such a distance, as Menzies Lyth pointed out, was a survival mechanism for nurses as there is a limit to the amount of suffering and pain one can cope with. The current view of nursing does not mean becoming so involved in people's lives that there is no longer a difference between people cared for as patients and one's own friends and relatives. Rather, it advocates a middle way, which involves the ability to come alongside people and get a real sense of what is going on for them. It also includes being able to empathise at a deep level, while at the same time having a clear sense that patients' lives and ours are quite separate.

This is, however, a skill that needs to be developed. Particularly for novice nurses, but also for the more experienced among us, it is not always easy to leave the patients 'at the door' when we go off duty. Metaphorically speaking, many nurses probably carry their patients around with them all the way home and sometimes perhaps continue to carry them around on their days off.

The more personal way many nurses now want to care for people is one of the reasons for the interest in supervision. Indeed, the restorative function is designed to provide support for nurses so that they can go on caring. It is now recognised that working with distressed, ill and dying people is in fact 'emotional labour'. In other words, it takes its toll unless we are supported ourselves. So first of all, the supportive function of clinical supervision helps us to offload the emotional stresses of our work.

However, if nursing is a therapeutic activity in its own right and we primarily use ourselves as part of that therapy, it is important that we know ourselves, in order to avoid inadvertently upsetting people, or judging or labelling them due to our own values and prejudices. Supervision therefore offers a supportive environment in which we can explore with a skilled facilitator our own thoughts, feelings, attitudes, values and norms as they affect our work. In other words, supervision is a way in which we can get to know ourselves better by developing and increasing our level of self-awareness.

During supervision we may, for example, examine our way of relating to a certain patient or colleague, or reflect on the meaning of a particular experience. We may want to ask ourselves questions such as 'what do I feel about this?', 'what does this mean to me?', 'when have I felt like this before?', 'what was the issue then?' or 'what is the common factor?'

In talking about specific people or situations, we may become aware of how the work is affecting us and how in turn we may be affecting others. As well as providing support, supervision is therefore also about learning about ourselves and about others. Through guided reflection we learn to see ourselves more clearly in relation to other people and how we function in practice. As nursing is in essence a people-oriented occupation, it is important to be aware of how we function interpersonally so that we can be 'the nurse we want to be' in all situations. We all have blind spots, areas where we function less effectively, perhaps because we feel uncomfortable or are unsure of how to behave. Supervision helps us to look at ourselves and find those blind spots, illuminate the dark corners and discover the areas where we want to develop further.

The learning that takes place through supervision is very different from the learning we experienced at school or, if we were trained some time ago, during our professional education. It is believed that adults have a different approach to learning than children. Adult learning is often called andragogy as opposed to pedagogy. According to the andragogical approach, adults learn best when they are actively involved in the learning process, when they decide what they want to learn and how best to go about it. In other words, adult learning involves taking responsibility for ourselves and the learning process (Knowles 1978).

Activity

Take some time to reflect on your work. It may be useful to visualise yourself going through a typical day, starting with getting ready to go to work, arriving, receiving hand-over, all the activities you carry out during your shift … giving hand-over, going home.
Really look at yourself in detail – how are you doing?
What would you like to know more about?
What interests you?
What do you find difficult to understand, hard to bear or to do?
What skills would you like to improve?
What new skills would you like to learn?

People are often surprised at the number and range of their answers to these questions, even if they have been functioning in a particular area for quite a while. This is because most of us do not habitually look at ourselves in such detail, but get used to seeing people and the world around us in a particular way. However, when we go on holiday to a place where we have never been before we see everything with unbiased eyes, so that everything looks very fresh. It is this type of unbiased looking that supervision seeks to develop, and why it is so useful to be guided while doing so. It often takes an outsider to point something out to us that we have long stopped seeing, which is why it may be preferable to have a supervisor who does not work in the same area as ourselves.

We have all been in situations (or know people who have been) where, for example, we were doing up a house and found that certain jobs took longer than others. After a while, however, we no longer saw that one wall needed another coat of paint, or that there was no light shade in the spare bedroom. A couple I once knew got stuck renovating a house and managed not to have a floor in the lounge for several years, having got used to living in the kitchen. It is only when people who had not visited them for a while commented on the lack of a floor that they'd say 'oh yes, I suppose we should do something about it some day'. If they are like another couple that comes to mind they probably never will, unless they want to sell the house. There is nothing like selling a house to make us look at it afresh, with the eyes of one who has not seen it before, critically, appraising, comparing.

In a way, supervision is like that. Imagine that you and the way you work are like a house that is for sale. Would anyone want to buy you, are you an attractive proposition, what price are you worth? Are you likely to get the price you want? Are improvements necessary? What would make you more attractive? In short, what could you do that would make people say 'Oh yes, I want that one'.

This kind of exercise is a useful one to do prior to commencing supervision as it will give you some ideas as to what you would like to achieve. It is useful to translate your ideas into some concrete goals and objectives which you can discuss with your prospective supervisors. Having thought about supervision beforehand and being clear regarding your personal aims will greatly facilitate its effectiveness. The exercise is also helpful prior to individual sessions. It is a good idea to bring a specific issue, problem or area of practice to supervision that has been thought about beforehand, and to know what is wanted from the session.

Working as a nurse often means having to take quick decisions or cope with difficult situations. In the context of supervision, self-awareness therefore involves reflecting on how we function professionally by becoming more conscious of how we think, feel and learn, and how we are perceived by others. In order to facilitate the growth of self-awareness, a supervisor may ask questions such as: 'How did you do that? What was your thinking behind that particular action? How did you feel when you were doing that? What do you think other people made of it?'

Ultimately, supervision is concerned with helping to develop clarity regarding such questions as: Who am I? How do I think, feel and act? – with reference to the person, the work, the hospital or other employing institution, society at large (de Vries-Geervliet 1992: 31). Clearly these are searching questions which are not answered lightly. Being honest, particularly with ourselves, is therefore a first requirement. Ofman identified the usefulness of identifying our 'core qualities', the tendencies that make us the people we are (Ofman 1995). According to Ofman, core qualities are central to the (core of) the person, tend to colour all other characteristics and are essentially an expression of the self.

Examples of core qualities are decisiveness, orderliness, the ability to put oneself in another's shoes, flexibility, and so on. It is important to realise that although central to the core of the person, core qualities are not static characteristics. Rather they are possibilities or tendencies which can be enhanced in the same way that the sound of a radio can be enhanced by tuning in correctly (Ofman 1995: 32). Core qualities should not be confused with skills, as they originate from within the person, whereas skills have been acquired. So whereas skills can be learnt, qualities can be developed.

Ofman (1995) further points out that if core qualities can be enhanced and developed positively, it follows that they can also be developed in a negative way by becoming distorted or exaggerated, thus turning a strength into a weakness. In everyday language we call this 'too much of a good thing' (p. 35). For example, a tendency to be helpful can turn into behaving like a busybody, whereas being easy-going may develop into laziness. So a core quality is like a coin, its strength is on one side, its distortion or trap on the other. It is two-way traffic: the core quality may lead to the distortion, but conversely the strength may be developed through giving attention to the distortion. We all like to present ourselves 'sunny side up', but every fried egg has two sides. So the distortion is an exaggeration rather than an opposite. That is how a strength can become a weakness and a weakness a strength.

When confronting people with a distortion, it is important to do this by focusing on the behaviour rather than the person (Ofman 1995: 36), so people are seen as positive in themselves, and it is only the distorted behaviour that is being focused on (Rogers 1961).

Activity

For this activity, it would be good to find another person who knows you quite well, and who is interested in developing self-awareness too. First help each other identify and list some core qualities – see if you can list at least five. Next, identify the exaggeration of the core qualities, the 'too much of a good thing', which represent the 'traps'.

If the exaggeration is not an opposite, what is the opposite of a core quality? According to Ofman, it is its allergy, the kind of things we cannot stand in other people and are in a manner of speaking 'allergic to'. Allergies have a tendency to let us fall into our traps. For example, if Graham's core quality is decisiveness, then passivity, or the inability of people to make a decision, will irritate him tremendously and is likely to lead him to decide for people – in other words, his allergy to passivity can let him fall into his trap of being bossy.

Ofman calls the way out of a trap the 'challenge'. For Graham not to fall into his trap of bossiness, he needs to exercise patience, which is the challenge for the core quality of decisiveness (Ofman 1995: 38–40). Thus every core quality has its positive and negative sides as well as its allergy and challenge. Once we identify our core qualities we can work out the other three factors and identify what we need to develop and what to watch out for. What the discovery of our core qualities shows is that strengths and weaknesses are essentially interrelated. Therefore the identification of core qualities is important. It does not imply a value judgement, simply a 'this is how it is, now how can I work with this?'

Activity

Go back to the list you made earlier and help each other identify the other three aspects of each of your core qualities. Having found them, discuss how they affect the way you work, if you want to, you can also discuss how they impinge on the rest of your life.
It may be useful to reflect on these two exercises in your journal.

The two activities above are very challenging as it is not easy to be confronted with traps and allergies. However, it is important not to see them as negative qualities, but as areas for development. Conversely, for many people, particularly women, it is easier to admit to negative qualities than strengths – therefore being confronted with positive qualities can be equally challenging. What these exercises are about is self-knowledge; it is only when we are aware of ourselves, our strengths and weaknesses and how these impinge on the way we work and interact with others, that we can start developing ourselves in a positive way. A skilful supervisor is an ideal ally in this process, which ultimately is about becoming more effective as a nurse. As pointed out above, nursing is essentially a therapeutic use of self, so the more aware we are of ourselves, the more conscious we will be in our interactions with people, and the more effective our work is likely to be.

As part of the preparation for supervision, it is of benefit to carry out exercises with others so that talking about ourselves and our work in a reflective way becomes more and more comfortable.

Activity

This exercise is once again for two people, taking turns at the roles of supervisor and supervisee. In the role of the supervisee, you talk about a situation in work when you were confronted with your allergy. What happened? The other person, in the role of supervisor, helps you to identify exactly what you did, the effect this had on the other person, and how you then felt. In other words, the person in the role of supervisor helps you to be precise and concrete about all aspects of the situation.

Having described the situation clearly, the 'supervisor' then helps the supervisee identify the strength (core quality) and the challenge and possibly also the allergy. It would be useful to then discuss how you could handle the situation better with the use of your challenge.

The above exercise was designed to begin to get a flavour of what is involved in supervision and the work that is involved for the supervisee. Although the supervisor needs to be skilled in helping the supervisee reflect on herself as well as how she works, the supervisee is the person who has to do the actual reflection. This requires honesty and the ability to take on board new insights about ourselves which may not always be comfortable. In the next section, I will discuss the skills needed by the supervisee in order to make effective use of the supervisory process.

IDENTIFYING SUPERVISORY NEEDS

Activity

Before becoming involved in supervision, you may like to ask yourself the following questions. It may be good to stop at this point, reflect on each question and note the answers in your reflective journal.
1. What do I want and need from supervision?
2. How do I choose a supervisor?

There is evidence to suggest that many potential supervisees are unsure as to what to expect from supervision, indeed some people are still uncertain after two years of regular supervision (Carroll 1996: 4). This is clearly an undesirable state of affairs but is possibly due to training courses giving attention to the role of the supervisor rather than that of the supervisee.

When I ask potential supervisees what they want and need, their answers tend to be remarkably similar and include support, a listening ear, help, someone to thrash problems out with, challenge, a different perspective, advice and new ideas. Looking at the identified needs more closely, the three functions of supervision as identified by Proctor (1988): 'restorative (supportive), educative, normative' are clearly identifiable. 'Support' and 'a listening ear' are obviously restorative, whereas 'someone to thrash out problems with' and 'challenge' would appear to fit under the normative heading, with the educative function being represented by 'help', 'advice' and 'a different perspective'.

Regarding the question of how to choose a supervisor, people are often at a loss. As supervision is still a relatively new concept, many people do not know how to go about this. However, being clear on what is wanted from supervision is a good starting point. A logical next step would be to look for a person likely to provide these needs. Before doing so, however, it is necessary to become more specific, as simply stating 'I need someone who can provide a different perspective' may not be sufficient. 'A different perspective from what?' and 'How will you know whether a person can provide it?' are good questions to ponder on. The following activities are designed to help focus the choice of supervisor.

Activity

Imagine that you are looking for a person to act as your supervisor. How do you want this person to be? Make a list of the relevant skills and attitudes you would like this person to have.

Then, for each item on the list, make a scale from 1 to 5, 1 representing low and 5 representing high, and place a cross where you would be most comfortable. In other words, if you wrote on your list of attitudes that you would like your supervisor to be challenging, how challenging would that be? Clearly if your answer to that is 5 you would look for a different person than if your answer is 2.

The above activity is essentially concerned with identifying the style of supervision that you would be most comfortable with. However, supervision is not just about being comfortable. As the previous section on core qualities may have made clear, supervision can often be uncomfortable and challenging. In other words, if you want to grow and develop, a certain amount of discomfort is unavoidable. However, it is up to each individual person to decide which particular style would be most beneficial for him or her at any particular time.

In addition to being clear on the preferred supervisory style, sharing a similar view on nursing is also an important consideration in making a choice of supervisor. For example, it would clearly be unhelpful for a Macmillan nurse engaged in helping the dying and bereaved to choose as a supervisor someone who mainly focuses on technology and who sees psychological and emotional care as an optional extra. It would therefore be helpful to first clarify one's own views on certain issues before discussing those with a potential supervisor.

Activity

The following questions are designed to help you clarify for yourself how you see the role of the nurse in general, and yourself in particular.

1. What is your definition of nursing?
2. What model or theory of nursing reflects your own view of what nursing is about?
3. What kind of a nurse are you?
4(a) If colleagues were asked to describe you as a nurse, what might they say?
  (b) What would you like them to say?
5(a) If patients were asked to describe you as a nurse, what might they say?
  (b) What would you like them to say?

Having completed the above questions and reflected on them in your journal, it may be good to discuss them with another person. The knowledge and insights gained will be useful in helping you decide what kind of person you would find beneficial as a supervisor. You may decide that you would like to work with someone who has views similar to yours. On the other hand, sometimes it can be challenging to choose someone who sees the role of the nurse differently, as this may force you to look at how you are working in greater depth.

If there was a discrepancy in your answers to the (a) and (b) parts of questions 4 and 5, you may want to choose a supervisor who comes close to the way you would like to be. On the other hand, if you choose someone whom you greatly admire, there could be a danger that you would simply copy them, which would be disempowering. A good supervisor will not let a supervisee fall into this trap, as he would realise that everyone has to develop their own way of working. What is right for one person does not necessarily rest easily with another.

In other words, the person you decide to choose as a supervisor will be someone who you feel you can work with, who can help you develop in certain areas and whose view of nursing is not so dissimilar that you do not talk the same language. Also, if you want to deepen your knowledge of your particular specialism, you may wish to choose a supervisor with relevant experience. If, on the other hand, your concerns in supervision tend to be more generic and not specific to the area in which you work, the supervisor's specialism may not be all that important. Furthermore, as discussed previously, someone from a different area, specialism or even discipline can often help to provide a clearer and wider perspective.

Other considerations regarding choice of supervisor concern more personal aspects such as gender, age or cultural background. As we saw in Chapter 2 (pp. 36–40), these are relevant factors which can impinge on the supervision process and which you therefore need to think about. You also need to think about when and where you would wish to see a supervisor. If you feel you can only commit yourself to supervision within your working hours this will clearly limit your choice of the people available. If, on the other hand you can be more flexible, you could choose to have supervision from someone who does not necessarily work for the same employer, thus greatly increasing your choice.

Once you have decided on the kind of person you are looking for, you need to approach suitable candidates in order to ascertain firstly, whether they are available for supervision, and secondly to see whether the two of you can actually work together. It is advisable not to narrow your list down to one person but to approach two or three people and have an exploratory conversation with each. If, on meeting, you feel too uncomfortable with the person, or that your views on nursing and on supervision are simply too divergent, it is important to say so and not to feel that now you have met, you have to embark on supervision. In any case, the choice is two-way, and the supervisor equally has a say in whether or not he feels that he can work with you.

When discussing the aspect of choice with nurses, I find that they are often amazed as they tend to assume that they will be told who to receive supervision from. However, unless supervision is managerial, choice of supervisor tends to be an accepted fact in the counselling and therapy world, as it is recognised that if people do not really wish to work together, then the supervision is unlikely to be very effective. Some organisations increase choice for supervisees by publishing a list of everyone prepared to take on the role of supervisor with a short description of themselves and how they like to work. It is then up to supervisees to make their choice and arrange an exploratory interview. As was discussed in Chapter 2 (pp. 41–42), a serious discussion is necessary in any case in order to draw up a contract. Also, having made your choice, there is no need to feel that you have to be supervised by this person for ever more. Included in the contract should be regular evaluation and recontracting, so that if either supervisee or supervisor feels that he or she would like a change, the contract can be terminated.

Activity

Imagine that you have made your provisional choice of supervisor and have arranged a meeting to discuss how the two of you will work together. Prior to this meeting you have agreed to think about your role as a supervisee. In other words, you need to draw up a list of what you need to do, i.e. your responsibilities, as well as what skills and attitudes might be helpful for you to really benefit from supervision.

Responsibilities will include some obvious factors such as being committed, not only turning up, but turning up on time, having prepared for the session, knowing what to bring to talk about, what your aims are in bringing that particular issue, as well as your supervisory needs in general. Some supervisors like to contract for the supervisee to keep a reflective journal and to bring relevant extracts of this to the session. From this, it follows that supervision does not just take place in the session. Indeed, Casement (1990) writes about the 'internal supervisor'. This means that, ideally, reflection is continuous and takes place 'in action' as well as 'on action', so that the supervision process starts before you even walk into the room (Schon 1983).

Having decided on the kind of person you would most like to work with in supervision, it is useful to look at yourself again in order to be clear on what you would like to get out of supervision. Bringing your work to supervision means a willingness to be genuine, to be honest about your thoughts, feelings and actions, and to be open to any challenges or different interpretations. Conversely, as supervision is essentially an exchange between equals, it also means being able to tell your supervisor if his approach is not helpful.

Activity

Answer the following questions and reflect on them in your journal. Regarding supervision:

1. What relevant skills do I have?
2. What relevant skills do I need to develop?

The skills that a supervisee needs in order to make the most of supervision may be grouped under the three functions: formative, supportive and normative (Proctor 1988; see Box 3.1).

Comparing your answers with those listed in Box 3.1 should give an indication of what skills you may need to develop, although you may well have thought of others not mentioned. In a nutshell, you need to be able to discuss an issue, problem or patient you are nursing in supervision and to have some idea why you are doing this. For example, you may want to reflect on how you have handled a certain situation because you were not happy with your performance, or you may just feel uneasy when nursing someone, but without knowing why. In the latter case, wanting to gain some clarity on why you feel like that would be the focus of the supervision.

It follows that you need to be very honest about how you work, what you think and what you feel. Pretending to be a different person from the one you are will serve no purpose and is, in any case, likely to get picked up sooner or later by the supervisor. It will also be necessary to be open to any feedback, positive as well as negative in order to help you develop further.

Box 3.1 Supervisee skills

Formative:	express feelings
clarify	being honest
analyse	
reflect	*Normative:*
verbalise	describe clearly
think	accept responsibility
	develop insight
Supportive:	self-awareness
accept support	action planning
accept praise	evaluate
accept positive criticism	accept criticism regarding areas for
relationship building	development
ability to trust	prioritise
being aware of feelings	

Clearly, being supervised is hard work, but it is also rewarding. Having someone focus on you and your work in a positive way is a real luxury and can be very enjoyable. In the next section, I will discuss how to prepare yourself so that you can get the best out of a session.

HOW TO PREPARE FOR A SUPERVISION SESSION

How you prepare for a session will to some extent depend on what you and your supervisor have already decided. Some people decide to set an agenda beforehand so that both supervisor and supervisee know what will be discussed in a particular session; others are happy to leave it more open. You will have to decide what feels most helpful for you. For example, you may decide to take a long, hard look at your practice and identify a number of areas you want to look at in depth. With your supervisor, you may decide how much time to devote to each area and what you would like to achieve as a result. If you do decide to take this approach it would be good to build in a proviso that you can change the topic should something more urgent crop up. If for example, you are having to handle an unusually difficult situation in work, you may like to use your next supervision session to reflect on this. Box 3.2 sets out the kind of topics people may discuss in supervision.

Box 3.2   Topics people may bring to supervision

- a theme
- a specific issue/problem/incident
- a specific area of practice (without there necessarily being a problem)

What supervision offers:
- an opportunity to look at one's practice with a fresh eye
- the benefit of someone else's perspective

Keeping a reflective diary is helpful when receiving supervision. Some people like to jot down their thoughts, feelings and preoccupations after every shift, whereas others prefer to do this on a weekly basis. We are often so busy that we do not find the time to reflect, and we forget what we are doing from one day to the next. However, a diary will give you something to start with as it will remind you what has been happening since the last time you had supervision. It may well be that reading through it you will discover recurring themes that need addressing. Doing a preliminary reflection prior to supervision may help you to pinpoint your concerns more precisely and thus help make the actual supervision session more effective.

Therefore, whether or not you decide the agenda beforehand, it is a good idea to give some thought first of all to what you want to discuss in your next session and, secondly, what your reason is for doing so. In addition, it may be helpful to use the three functions of supervision (formative, normative and supportive) as a framework to decide on your aims for the session.

For example, imagine that you find it difficult to speak up at team meetings. You may find that 'not knowing how to get your voice heard' is in fact a 'theme' emerging from your journal. Perhaps you found that you were not listened to in a meeting recently. You thought you had made a relevant point or useful suggestion, but somehow it got overlooked.

In preparation for the supervision session, it would be useful to describe such an experience in some detail, so that you and your supervisor can use it as a prototype to analyse, reflect on and work with. Also, prior to the supervision session, you may like to think about the kind of role you do wish to play in a team or a meeting. Are you perhaps a frustrated leader or do you want to be a more useful team member? Useful questions to ask yourself include:

- What exactly happened? (normative and supportive functions)
- How did you try to make your point? (normative and supportive functions)
- What or who prevented it from being heard? (normative and supportive functions)
- What did you do then? (normative and supportive functions)
- How did you feel? (supportive function)
- What questions arise for you from this situation? (educative function)
- What is it that you feel you need to learn? (educative function)

Being able to describe and conceptualise an issue in this way is a useful skill and will become easier the more it is practised. After a while, people tend to find that for some issues that they used to have problems with, this kind of personal reflection is sufficient to provide answers. However, many other more complex issues and situations are difficult to unravel alone and are better dealt with in supervision.

The next two activities are designed to help you practise preparing for a supervision session.

Activity

Imagine that you are a community nurse who has been looking after Jim for a few months. Jim is in his mid-thirties, married to Joanna, and they have two young children. Three years ago, Jim was diagnosed with lung cancer and treated accordingly. A few months ago it was realised that the cancer had returned and Jim is once again receiving treatment. You talked about Jim in your last supervision session as you had been feeling some vague concern which you could not put your finger on. During the course of the session you came to realise that you had not seen Joanna for a while, as she is either not at home or on the verge of going out when you call. Meanwhile, Jim has been putting a brave face on things. He was very positive a few years ago, but does not seem quite himself lately. You have not really had a good talk with him and have the feeling that he is keeping the conversation at a superficial level. You decide to make Jim and Joanna the focus of your next supervision session. What will you want to reflect on? (normative function) What do you need help with? (educative function) What do you need support for? (supportive function)

You may choose to reflect on how you approach Jim when you see him. In order to make matters less abstract, it can be useful to take five minutes out of the last time you saw him and describe these in detail. You can either write it out beforehand or perhaps act the situation out in the session with the supervisor. The important thing is that you have thought about it prior to the session. In doing this, it may become clear that you have been colluding with Jim in keeping matters at a superficial level. Perhaps you sense that he is deeply troubled about something, but you are afraid that you may not be able to help him. At the same time, you are not happy as you know that you want to do more but what you need help with is how to go about it. In supervision you may like to discuss strategies for finding out how Jim really feels and whether he would like to talk with you. The fact that Joanna is always out or about to go out may also need addressing; perhaps she is avoiding you, in which case you may need to find out why. Being able to talk about a case such as this as well as developing ways of handling it is in itself supportive. However, it may well be that once you develop a more open and honest relationship with both Jim and Joanna, they tell you what is really troubling them. They may be afraid of death or have sexual problems, for example, which you may find difficult to cope with, in which case, being able to offload in supervision becomes even more important.

Activity

This activity is a little different as it encourages you to look at a patient from her perspective, which can be a very helpful way of reflecting as it may give you an indication of how you can really help her. While reading it try and imagine that you are the patient. Take some time to get into the situation.

The name of the patient is Yvonne; she is 42 and waiting for surgery. This is her story.

'When my doctor first told me that I had cancer I was furious. I felt that it wasn't fair – I had always looked after myself. I have never smoked, exercise regularly – three times a week, I mean, I swim, go to aerobics and do weights! I eat a healthy diet. OK, I have a glass of wine from time to time, but nothing outrageous, and anyway it is supposed to be good for you isn't it?

I have always been fitter than most women my age and I often get compliments on my looks. I have always had a good body and enjoyed men looking at me. It's just one of those things I'd always been used to. When Frank and I got divorced five years ago, I went out with quite a few men in the first year or so. So, I suppose I'd always taken my body and being attractive for granted.

But now I feel betrayed, confused. How can I have breast cancer? It's such a horrible, alien thing, growing inside me. The doctor thinks that the operation will be successful and that he can remove the cancer. But you can never be sure can you? I don't feel that I can ever trust my body again. And as for a sex life, well, I suppose I can forget that. What man is going to want me now? I am not in a relationship at the moment, so I don't have anyone to support me. And I have needs! It may be strange, but I feel desperate sometimes for a man's strong arms around me, someone to cuddle up to in bed. I miss that more than sex at the moment, although that has always been important too. But I suppose I'll have to forget about that now, it's so unfair, I'm not old, but I feel that I shall be condemned to live as though I'm 70. And I'm so, so frightened.'

Now take 10 minutes or so to write in your journal anything that comes into your mind. Do not edit out anything, just write whatever comes into your head. How are you (as Yvonne) feeling? What do you want? What do you not want? How can your primary nurse help?

Then, as yourself, read this reflection and imagine that you are Yvonne's primary nurse. How prepared do you feel to help Yvonne with her needs? What needs have you identified that you do not know how to meet? Perhaps you feel unsure about how to help Yvonne, or maybe you have some ideas but want to discuss them with someone first. You may feel that you want to talk with Yvonne but then feel pressurised to 'do something' but you do not know what. All these are legitimate concerns to talk about in supervision. At this stage, it is useful to determine how your supervisor can help, and what outcome you would like from your next supervision session.

As Yvonne's primary nurse, you may find looking after her very difficult, perhaps because she is the same age as you, or because you have lost someone you were close to due to breast cancer. As nurses, we tend to think that with our uniform we put on a professional persona and leave all our personal worries and problems behind. However laudable that may be, we are still the same person and the work will affect us, however much we try and prevent this. It tends to be more helpful to be aware of how the work affects us then to try and pretend it is not happening. For example, to continue with the hypothetical scenario, you may find it difficult to work with Yvonne but not realise why. All you know is that you seem to try and get others to care for her and that she makes you feel uncomfortable. However, at the same time, you know that you are not doing a good job for her and that she is not receiving the care she should. Knowing that is enough to take to supervision. Your supervisor may ask you to reflect on exactly what it is that you find so difficult. She could even role play Yvonne, ask you how you feel and give you feedback on how you made her (in her role as Yvonne) feel. It might be, for example, that your mother died of breast cancer when you were young, but you had imagined that you had got over it and that it no longer affected you. Realising that it does affect you is in itself helpful, a problem we are not afraid to look squarely in the eye is already half solved. Knowing now how looking after a patient with breast cancer affects you, you are in a position to discuss with your supervisor what would be helpful for you as well as Yvonne. Not only is all this tremendously supportive, the normative function is also obvious as the quality of Yvonne's care is involved. Lastly, finding out more about yourself is also educative as you have learnt a bit more about yourself, thus supervision can promote continuous personal as well as professional growth.

REFLECTING ON THE SUPERVISION SESSION

Having received supervision, it is useful to keep an account of what happened in the session in your reflective journal (de Vries-Geervliet 1992: 19–21). We suggest that you not only record the facts but also reflect on the session. The following are questions that may be used as a guide for the keeping of such a record:

- What happened in the session?
- What was your experience?
- How did you feel during the session?
- How did you feel afterwards?
- What did your supervisor do?
- What worked?
- What did not work?
- What did you do?

- How did you respond to your supervisor's questions or suggestions?
- Were your goals fulfilled?
- What new insights did you gain?
- How will you integrate these new insights into your practice?
- What action, if appropriate, did you decide to take? When and how?

As stated earlier, being a supervisee is an excellent preparation for becoming a supervisor, particularly if sessions are reflected on in this way. Making the supervision process clear, conscious and above board will greatly enhance its effectiveness.

CONCLUSION

In this chapter, it has been demonstrated that preparation for supervision is important, not just for the supervisor but also for the supervisee. Becoming aware of how we work as well as knowing our strengths and weaknesses is a first requisite for supervision. The ability to reflect, aided by a journal or diary as well as supervision will help with our continuous professional as well as personal development, which in itself is likely to lead to greater job satisfaction. Also, as has been pointed out, receiving supervision is a very good way of preparing oneself for the role of supervisor, which is the topic of the next chapter.

REFERENCES

Benner P, Wrubel J 1989 The primacy of caring: stress and coping in health and illness. Addison-Wesley, Menlo Park, CA
Boud D, Keogh R, Walker D 1985 Reflection: turning experience into learning. Kogan Page, London
Carroll M 1996 Counselling supervision. Cassell, London
Casement P 1990 Further learning from the patient. The analytic space and process. Routledge, London
de Vries-Geervliet L 1992 Voorbereiden op supervisie. H. Nelissen, Baarn
Halldorsdottir S 1991 Five basic modes of being with another. In Gaut D A, Leininger M M (eds) Caring: the compassionate healer. Center for Human Caring, National League for Nursing Press, New York, p. 37–50
Knowles M 1978 The adult learner: a neglected species, 2nd edn. Gulf, Houston, TX
Menzies Lyth E E P 1988 The functioning of social systems as a defence against anxiety: a report on a study of the nursing service of a general hospital. In Menzies Lyth I. Containing anxiety in institutions. Free Association Books, London, p 43–85

Ofman D 1995 Bezieling en kwaliteit in organisaties, 2nd edn. Servire, Cothen
Proctor B 1988 Supervision: a working alliance. Alexia, Sussex
Richardson G, Maltby H 1995 Reflection-on-practice: enhancing student
    learning. Journal of Advanced Nursing 22: 235–242
Rogers C R 1961 On becoming a person. Houghton Mifflin, Boston
Schon D A 1983 The reflective practitioner. Basic Books, New York
Watson J 1985 Nursing: human science and human care. A theory of nursing.
    Appleton-Century-Crofts, Norwalk, CT

4

Becoming a supervisor

Supervisors can only take others to a depth of exploration and reflection that they have personally and professionally experienced themselves. (Long & Chambers 1996)

In order to help supervisees reflect openly and honestly on themselves and their practice, supervisors need to be able to do so too. In other words, they need to know what it is like to be at the receiving end of supervision. Also, as nursing is now recognised as involving the use of self in a therapeutic manner, that 'self' needs to be up to it, so a certain amount of self-awareness and self-exploration is essential. However, as is clear from the above quotation, supervisors will only be able to help their supervisees to engage in such a process if they have also looked at themselves and how they use themselves in their work. This is because a person with only limited self-awareness is unlikely to be able to help others discover things about themselves that they do not already know.

This chapter is in two parts. In the first section, the focus is on some essential supervisory skills, after which the self-development of supervisors is discussed. As in Chapter 3, I recommend keeping a journal throughout the reading of the chapter in order to complete the activities and record any reactions to the material presented.

WHAT IS INVOLVED IN BECOMING A SUPERVISOR?

Some people may choose to become a supervisor because they see it as a challenge and a natural progression in their working career. Others may find themselves being asked by potential supervisees whether they are interested, which may be experienced as flattering and a recognition of one's worth as a nurse. It is not uncommon, however, for people to react with a feeling of panic and to wonder what exactly is involved and whether they will be able to cope. Yet others may be told by their managers that supervision is going to be part of their role, in which case it would not be surprising to react with apprehension or even some resistance.

Whichever way people come to the role of supervisor, it is likely to be experienced as a demanding and challenging, yet ultimately very rewarding role. Before continuing, please stop for a moment and complete the following activity.

Activity

If you are not already supervising, imagine that you have decided to accept an invitation to become a supervisor. Take 10 minutes or so to ponder on the question 'What do I want to get out of being a supervisor?' Note your answers in your journal.

The reasons people have for taking on the role of supervisor very greatly. You might feel initially that it offers you some welcome time out from your job, or think that it will look good on your curriculum vitae and will therefore help you to advance your career. You may welcome the opportunity of learning a skill that is different from those you normally use. The idea of helping others to do their job well is also a common reason. Particularly once people have been supervising for a little while, they realise how much they learn themselves, as potentially every supervisee and every supervision session contains a valuable learning opportunity. They find that they learn about their own effectiveness as a supervisor and about how other people, work, function, think and react. Acting as a supervisor also offers the opportunity to learn a great deal about many aspects of nursing and to gain a wider view, particularly if supervisees come from outside your own area of work.

Above all, and perhaps unexpectedly, supervision offers a chance to learn about yourself. Honesty and a certain amount of self-exploration is essential if we are to avoid inadvertently harming others or using them to further our own ends. It is therefore important to be aware of the 'shadow side' of helping and the dangers of ego tripping (Hawkins & Shohet 1989: 8). After a good session it is easy to pat yourself on the back and think 'aren't I a good facilitator, look what I have just done'. It can be seductive to bask in this glory and to let others as well as ourselves think that we are something special, somehow a cut above the rest. In reality, however, to be really helpful, all we can ever do is to 'keep open the space in which people can learn and grow' and to be the 'servants of the process' (Hawkins & Shohet 1989: 9).

Part of becoming a supervisor therefore involves being honest about your motives and seeing them for what they are. It is not in itself wrong to feel the need to be valued and to be recognised for doing a good job; these are needs that we all share. What can be dangerous is their denial. If you are not honest with yourself and deny those needs, it can lead you to use others to make yourself feel better. Rather than facilitating others to work out their own problems, you may take over and tell them what to do, make them feel bad, or tell them how brilliantly you coped in a similar situation. This may make you feel good, but is unlikely to do much for the self-esteem and development of the supervisee.

So if you do find yourself somehow using a supervision situation for your own ends, it is useful to stop and think 'What is going on here?', 'Why am I doing this?'. It may well be that there is a lack of recognition in other areas of your life, in which case you may need to do something about that. Also, as with all helping-type roles, in becoming a supervisor, it is essential to ensure that you have an effective support system for yourself. Ideally, therefore, every supervisor would have supervision herself for all aspects of her own job, which would naturally also include supervision for her supervisory role.

Having gained an idea of what you personally would like to get out of being a supervisor, it is time to look at what it is you will need in order to fulfil that function. For this you will need to be clear on what supervision is, what it is for, and how well prepared you feel to take on the role.

Activity

In your journal write a paragraph in answer to each of the following questions:

- What is supervision?
- What is the purpose of supervision?
- What does the role of supervisor entail?
- What relevant skills do I possess?

- What relevant skills do I need to develop?
- What other training needs do I have?

Ultimately, supervision is about helping workers to function well in all aspects of their job and to facilitate their continuing growth and development. Whichever aspect of the job is under scrutiny, in the final analysis, the aim of supervision is to provide an optimum service for the users of that service, which means that it also contains a quality control element. However, that control is not exercised in a top-down, authoritative manner but by means of supporting the supervisee to critically reflect on his own practice, and to change and improve that practice when required.

Thus supervision involves challenge, support and empowerment, as well as the ability to stand back and to trust supervisees to come to their own conclusions and to take whatever action is necessary. Inevitably, being a supervisor also means acting as a role model, as the way in which you relate to the supervisee is likely to affect how the supervisee in turn relates to others. There is no getting away from this. Although elsewhere I have stressed the importance of maintaining equality in the supervisory relationship as much as possible, a certain authority is nevertheless inherent in the function of supervisor. It is this essential paradox that is so exiting and creative. The aim is to be egalitarian, while at the same time accepting the responsibility of the role and the awareness of its visibility. As a supervisee, you can be relatively anonymous; as a supervisor you are not. Without necessarily divulging the details of a session, supervisees will talk to each other about how helpful they find the experience and they are likely to compare notes regarding their supervisors' styles. Supervisors, on the other hand, are not free to do so as talking about their supervisees would constitute a breach of confidentiality. If supervisees found that they were being discussed by their supervisors they would very likely discontinue the process and go elsewhere.

So what are the skills required to act as a supervisor? Many of the skills that most nurses use as part of their everyday work are likely to be useful in supervision, such as meeting new people and building up a relationship with them, gaining someone's trust and cooperation, being with people in difficult and emotional situations, as well as supporting, guiding, prioritising and teaching. So rather than learning a whole range of new skills, what is needed is an adaptation, further development or fine tuning of the skills already in existence.

Listening

Most people, for example, place the ability to listen at the top of their list, but the extent to which they feel they already have this skill varies. In our experience, undergoing training for supervision can occasionally be a salutary experience. People who think they are good listeners can, on watching a video of themselves as supervisor, find that their self-image takes somewhat of a dent. Instead of really listening, they may jump to conclusions, interrupt or simply not hear what the other person is saying. In everyday life this is not wrong, but is simply how people tend to communicate. However, in the supervision context the normal everyday activity of listening gets used in a special way, involving an active process, rather than a passive 'taking in what someone is saying'.

First of all you need to really *hear* what someone is telling you, either consciously or inadvertently. This involves listening with your heart, mind and body. The terms 'free floating attention' or 'holistic listening' are useful descriptions of the very special type of listening involved. In order to do so, however, you must be still yourself, as you will not be able to give another person your full attention if you have your mind on other matters. That is why it is so important to have free, uninterrupted time for supervision as well as a quiet place. Fitting it in a quick half hour in the office will not work. Another word for being still within ourselves is 'being centred', which means finding a still, peaceful place within ourselves.

Activity

This is an exercise in centring. Read it through several times so that you are clear on what to do. Alternatively, you may like someone to read the instructions to you, or you could read them yourself and record them on a tape.

Find a quiet place where you can be alone for five minutes without being interrupted. Sit in a comfortable, ideally a straight-backed, chair, with your legs uncrossed, both feet on the floor and your hands resting loosely in your lap. When you feel ready, close your eyes and concentrate on breathing gently in and out. Try slowly counting to four while breathing in, hold it for two counts, and then breathe out for four, hold for two, and so on; do this three or four times. Then gradually let yourself become aware of your body. Mentally go through your body and note the position of every part of it, starting with your head and working your way down. Take your time while doing this and continue to breathe slowly to the same rhythm that you have established. Then notice whether you have tension anywhere in your body, focus your attention on it and let it go by repeating to yourself 'release and relax, release and relax', until you can feel the tension diminishing.

Become aware of the air against your skin, the feel of the chair against your back and bottom, the floor against your feet, and then focus on all the sounds you can hear. See if you can first concentrate on the sounds in the room in which you are sitting, before letting yourself hear any sounds coming from outside it. All the while continue to breathe in the easy rhythm you have established. Notice any thoughts that come into your mind, but do not dwell on them. Simply notice them for what they are and then let them go. Continue to sit like this, in full centred awareness for a few minutes more.

After a few minutes focus on the room in which you are sitting and then, once again, become aware of your body. Move your fingers and your toes, count slowly to three, and let your eyes open on the count of three. You may like to have a bit of a stretch and a yawn.

Although this is an exercise in awareness, most people find it really relaxing. That is because being centred is to be relaxed, no matter what is happening. Those of you who have done this kind of exercise before will recognise that the more often you practise it, the easier it gets, until you are able to centre yourself any time, anywhere. It is a particularly useful skill when you find yourself in a stressful or difficult situation, as it will help prevent you from being caught up in other people's emotions or panic. Naturally, in such cases, you may only have a few seconds rather than minutes, but once you are practised this will be enough.

Being able to listen to another person from a quiet, centred place is like being at the eye of a storm. No matter how wild the hurricane, at the centre everything is peaceful and quiet. Being at the eye of the storm, as it were, is clearly a useful thing to be able to do, not just in supervision, but also in your everyday working and personal life.

Having discussed the place from which to begin, we now turn our attention to the activity of holistic listening itself. In a way, a start has already been made, in that during centring we simply notice everything there is to notice with all our senses. We take note of what we hear and feel, as well as what is going on in our body and our mind. We do this not by focusing on it, but simply by noticing it. During listening we have our eyes open, so we add to it – everything that we see. It is good to practise centring and listening with eyes closed as often as possible, at least twice a day, to avoid all this information being swamped by what we take in through our eyes.

So when you listen to another person you listen first of all to the words, to what he is saying, what he is not saying and what you seem to be able to 'read between the lines'. Reading (or rather listening) between the lines and hearing what is not being said will involve taking in *how* someone is talking rather than *what* they are saying.

Is his tone of voice cheerful, sad, excited? Does he speak freely, or is he hesitant, leaving long gaps between sentences? How does he seem? What message are you getting from his facial expression, they way he looks at you (or avoids looking at you), the way he sits, the way he gestures, fidgets or swings his legs? All this non-verbal information needs to be attended to, as it is now generally recognised that what people tell us non-verbally has far more meaning than what they actually say. Try saying 'Where is Jenny?' in as many different ways as possible and you will see that the same three words can take on many different meanings. If you then add body movement and facial expression, the picture gets more complex still.

So far we have focused on what we can pick up directly from the other person. Another part of holistic listening, however, is to be aware of what is going on with yourself. How does being with the other person make you feel in your body? Do you suddenly feel tired or have butterflies which were not there before? Equally, your feelings and emotions provide another 'sense' which must also be attended to. The more practised you are at being still in yourself, the more likely you are to be able to pick up the subtle shifts and changes in the feelings in your body, indeed all your senses, as you listen.

Being still within yourself means that what you notice is likely to be something communicated by the other person. For example, while listening you may become aware of feeling sad, whereas you felt perfectly normal before and have no particular reason for feeling sad. It is likely that you are somehow picking up the other person's sadness, which he is communicating to you, albeit not in words. In Chapter 6 (pp. 170–179), which focuses on the process of supervision, I will discuss how to make use of all this information. For now, it may be useful for you to practise this type of listening in your everyday life, as you are talking with patients, or perhaps sitting with your friends in a pub.

As mentioned earlier, holistic listening is also called 'free floating attention' which expresses even more clearly its 'here-and-now' nature. In other words, you give another person your total attention, rather than focusing on only a small part of what they are communicating. This means that you attend to everything that is happening as it happens, in the here and now. Initially this may be difficult, but as you gain more experience as a supervisor, it becomes gradually easier to do, until you are likely to find yourself doing it without really trying.

Responding

So far we have concentrated on listening, which as we have seen is an active rather than a passive process. But there is more to communication than listening. For a start, you have to demonstrate that you are listening, by your posture, by looking at the other person and by responding. Minimally, you can encourage the other person to go on talking by nodding, grunting 'hmm, hmm', saying 'go on' or repeating the last few words. The latter should not be overdone, however, or you will be in danger of sounding like a parrot. Other active skills include paraphrasing, reflection and asking questions.

Paraphrasing involves saying back to the other person what he has just told you, but in a slightly different way, whereas reflection may go beyond the facts to include feelings that are being communicated non-verbally. Paraphrasing and reflection are helpful in that their use demonstrates to the supervisee that you are listening, but they also offer an opportunity to check out that you have understood what you are hearing. Leaving a margin for being corrected by saying something such as: 'Can I just stop you there? So what you are saying is … is that right?' This gives the supervisee an opportunity to correct you without feeling that you are not listening, as it is obvious that you really want to understand.

Finally, responding in this way from time to time helps you to concentrate and keep track of the information being given. Particularly when a supervisee is relating a complicated situation which has many feelings attached, it is helpful to respond actively in order to avoid being swamped. In a way, you are chunking the information given by the supervisee into bite-sized pieces for yourself.

Paradoxically, although you are basically feeding back to the supervisee what he has just told you, it has the effect of encouraging him to say more. Also, hearing someone else say what he has just said can sometimes in itself help him to see things more clearly.

Another useful skill is summarising which involves briefly saying 'in a nutshell' what the other person has been telling you. Thus it is quite possible to offer a summary of a few sentences after you have been talking with someone for 15 minutes. Summarising helps to make sense of the information. For example, you may get the impression that you have now heard all the facts of the situation and want to state them succinctly before deciding where you go from there. Other, more advanced skills involve the ability to challenge a person, or perhaps confront him with a difficult truth about himself, without hurting him in the process. In Chapter 6, I provide examples of how the skills mentioned can be used in the process of supervision.

Using emotions

Skilful supervision means making use of your emotions as well as your mind and your intelligence. In a way, being able to use the full gamut of your emotions skilfully is more important than being able to analyse brilliantly. This is because almost everything we do as nurses involves communication with other people, which means dealing with feelings and emotions. Although some may like to believe otherwise, when things go wrong between people it is rarely due to a fault in someone's intellectual capacity, but nearly always due to emotions: likes, dislikes, feelings of being mistreated, undervalued, exploited, and so on; the list can be endless. Therefore, in supervision it is useful to unravel the feeling of all those involved. Similarly, as supervision is in itself a relationship, it is important that the supervisor is able to use the range of feelings appropriately, not only for the benefit of the supervisory relationship itself, but also to act as a role model for the supervisee.

As a result of psychological research, seven main emotions have been identified, so-called sentic states, each with its own emotional rhythm (Clynes 1980). The seven states are awe, joy, eros, love, grief, anger and hate. Each state is believed to be located in a particular part of the body, which, for those of you interested in yoga, correspond to the seven chakras. Awe is located at the top of the head, joy in the middle of the forehead, eros at the area around the mouth and base of the throat, love in the heart, grief in the navel (solar plexus) area, anger in the genital area, and hate at the base of the spine (Clynes 1978).

Each sentic state has a positive as well as a negative facet. For example, anger can be expressed negatively, by completely losing one's temper and stomping about ineffectively, or positively, by simply stating one's case in an assertive manner. A good supervisor will use all sentic states positively and move freely between them. We all tend to have our own preferred ways of behaving, not all of which are helpful. If a supervision session gets stuck, for example, this may be due to each person being stuck in a sentic state. What is called for here is a change in rhythm by the supervisor. Instead of listening empathically and patiently waiting for the supervisee to come to the point, it may be helpful to shift gear completely and ask a controversial question, challenge the supervisee or change the topic entirely. (In the latter case it would be good to come back to it later, when it might well be that the original impasse has been resolved in the meantime.)

Activity

In your journal, write two paragraphs on the positive and negative aspects of each sentic state. What do they mean to you? Which ones do you feel comfortable with; which are difficult? To what extent are you able to use each state positively? Where are your areas of negativity?

It is important to be honest with yourself as this will give you valuable information regarding where you may need to do some work.

To be holistic nurses we must be comfortable with all aspects of what it means to be human. If supervision is to help us to develop the way we work and the way we care, it follows that getting in touch with all these sentic states is necessary.

Figure 4.1 sets out our development of each sentic state into a positive and negative expression as well as a lack of expression and any gender differences. It also indicates where the sentic states

Positive expression	Negative expression		Gender	Lack
Able to wonder, to be amazed, to give praise where due 'Gosh – you did that well' 'wow' (Receiving energy)	Paralysis Stupefaction – like a rabbit 'frozen' Hero worship	**Awe** (top of head)	Men more likely to be in awe of vastness	Feeling incompetent, low self esteem seeing other people as better Cynicism
Playfulness, delight, happy, enjoyment Enthusiasm Good at motivating others (playful energy)	Over the top Lack of consideration for others, or anything Overly excitable Out of control Lack of focus – all over the place	**Joy** (middle of forehead)	In our culture men having fun appears to be more acceptable	Depression No get up and go, low energy Bored
Sensitivity In touch with our body (The princess and the pea) Adaptability, fluidity (Giving out energy)	Over indulgence – food, drink, drugs, sex Addiction, craving, grasping attachment Mechanistic materialism or dislike of own body, masochism, asceticism, frugality, prudery	**Eros** (sensuality) (mouth, base of throat)	More acceptable for women to be sensitive and in touch with own bodies Tendency to be more expression of sensuality in women's clothing, more sensuous, touchable materials In our culture – touch between women more acceptable	Rigidity – rule bound Insensitivity to others and to own comfort Not in touch with own body

Figure 4.1   Sentic states and their expression.

are located in the body (Clynes 1980) and outlines the emotional expression associated with each one. The first column outlines positive expression of each state, with the second column describing a maladaptive, negative expression. The fourth column explains what happens if a person is not in touch with a particular sentic state, whereas the third column discusses possible differences between men and women in the way they experience and express the states. With regard to the latter, it is important to remember that these are generalisations only and that there is likely to be individual variation. For example, I postulate that men are more inclined to be in awe of vastness – of the universe, a mountain or a car – which does not mean that women cannot feel such awe too. It is just that, on the whole, men appear to have this tendency more often than women.

Positive expression	Negative expression		Gender	Lack
Caring, nourishing, giving, warm, helpful	Using others to meet own needs		Women generally more in touch with love	Overly focused on rationality, logic, 'the mind'
Healthy self esteem	Fear; over focusing on self, selfish and self-centred		Women also with the negative expression of self-sacrifice and self-denial	Lonely, difficulty in forming intimate relationships
Self acceptance, comfortable with self				
Liking and loving self	Focusing on sex rather than love – using others as sex objects	**Love** (heart)		Difficult to reach out, ask for help
Able to emotionally 'hold' others	Greed			Alienation
Able to accept others as they are	or			Feelings of unreality
Compassion, giving praise when due	Self-sacrifice; self-denial, uncritical			Judgemental
Generosity				Lack of self-love
(Giving out energy)				Perfectionism
A final loving message to the dead (Kurtz 1990: 126)	Inconsolable Stuck Useless suffering Unable to accept the loss	**Grief** (navel, solar plexus)	Men more likely to either deny or be inconsolable	Hard – harsh Lack of appreciation
Able to appreciate – permeability – openness	Denial Addiction to grief		In our culture it is more acceptable for women to express grief	Lack of understanding
(Letting in energy)				

Figure 4.1   (Cont'd).

You will already have some idea regarding your own feelings about each sentic state by completion of the previous activity. It is now time to become more specific and to identify where your personal learning points lie.

Activity

Have a good look at Figure 4.1. Now refer back to the paragraphs written for the previous activity, then place a cross in one of the sections for each sentic state to indicate which way of expression most accurately describes your own position.

As stated earlier, to be an effective supervisor you should be able to express each sentic state positively and move freely between each state as the occasion demands. However, very few of us are able to do this for every state. We all have areas of difficulty, where we have developed maladaptive expressions or no expression at all. Also, as is clear from Figure 4.1, there is a

Positive expression	Negative expression		Gender	Lack
Clean, clear in the moment, direct (this is what I feel now), appropriate target	Out of control, rage, violence, destructive, ineffective		In our society generally less tolerated for women – unless negatively	Difficulty with taking authority (e.g. chairing meeting, teaching)
Assertive – calm	Inappropriate target (displaced)		(Acting the victim, manipulative)	Being walked over, door mat
Authoritative, leadership	Confrontational			Feeling weak, insecure
Gives appropriate feedback	Combative	**Anger**		Sense of 'not being good enough'
Constructive criticism	Critical	(genital area)		Feeling a failure despite accomplishments
Able to challenge in a supportive manner	or Goes underground, acting the victim, manipulative			Craving security and safety
(Pushing through energy : an energy of transformation)				Fear of risk
Decisive – clean (cut like a knife)	Ruthless		Women often not sufficiently in touch with positive expression	Problems with boundaries and endings (difficulty in letting go and moving on)
Clear about own boundaries and able to stick to them	Lack of concern for the feelings of others Overly competitive		Women more often negatively by self-destructive behavior	Letting problems fester
Clear contracting	Unforgiving, ignorance, refusal to accept a fait accompli			Finding it difficult to throw things away
High self worth	or	**Hate**		Fear of separation
Able to let go of the past appropriately	Goes underground – turning inwards – self-destructive or manipulative behaviour	(base of spine)		Conservative, fearful of change
Able to live in the present – knowing that there is only the here and now				Inability to finish tasks, projects, relationships
Able to forgive and forget				Procrastination
(Cutting off or pushing away energy)				Workaholism

Figure 4.1 (Cont'd).

gender difference, possibly due to the different ways in which men and women are socialised. In our upbringing and in our lives generally, we need to experience all states positively in order to develop positive expression ourselves.

For example, a lack of love in early life, perhaps caused by an absent or preoccupied mother, can have the effect of causing one to lose contact with one's body and focus almost totally on the mind. This can have the effect of someone almost literally retreating 'to the confines of their mind', leading to 'the thinking mind ... becoming ... the locus of the sense of self' (Epstein 1996: 53). Since in our society, boys are encouraged to 'behave like men' meaning not crying or showing emotion, they may experience this as not getting the love and physical contact they need, which is perhaps why men in particular have a tendency to focus on the mind. Children tend to have less contact with their fathers than their mothers, and at a fairly early age, boys get the message that they must somehow become like this sometimes remote and unemotional figure. It is no accident that there are far more women in all the helping professions than men, although there are signs that the balance is beginning to shift somewhat as people become more aware, and it becomes more acceptable for men to be in touch with their emotions and to take on a caring role.

Unless you are an unusually fortunate person, in light of the above discussion, it is likely that you have placed a number of crosses in the 'negative expression' and 'lack of expression' columns. There is no need to be disheartened by this as becoming aware of our areas of difficulty is a first and necessary step towards doing something about it. The following activity is designed to help you become more comfortable with a positive expression of all the sentic states.

Activity

Some people like to do this activity on their own, whereas others prefer to do it with another person reading out the instructions. I suggest that it is a good idea to carry it out with someone else, preferably a person who you feel very comfortable with, so that you can talk about it afterwards. As this is a fairly penetrating exercise which may reveal some hitherto unknown truths about yourself, it would be good to have the support of another person, so choose wisely.

Decide which sentic state you wish to work on first. Begin by spending a few minutes doing the centring exercise outlined earlier, up to the point where you are aware of all sensations, sounds, feelings and thoughts. Next, focus on the chosen sentic state by continuing to breathe in the rhythm you have established and repeating in your mind the word depicting the state. For example, if you have chosen to work on hate, you say the word 'hate' in your mind and repeat it slowly six or seven times. Next, stop counting and note what is happening in your body. You may, for example, become aware of a feeling of nausea in your stomach or a slight increase in your heart rate.

Without changing your breathing just focus on whatever you are feeling and watch what happens. An image or memory may appear. Just look at it without trying to change it. If you are working with another person, it is helpful to talk about what you are experiencing as it happens. You may well find that the feelings or images slowly change as you focus on them.

When you feel that you have had enough, begin to breathe a little deeper, become aware of the whole of your body and of your surroundings, count slowly to three, and on the count of three open your eyes. It will be helpful to talk with the other person about your experience or write about it in your journal before doing anything else. In particular, you should ask yourself 'What is it I need to learn?'

If you have not done this kind of exercise before you may have found it difficult to relax into it. Do not worry, it will get easier the more often you do it. In any case, it is unlikely that carrying out the activity just once will solve whatever problem you have with the sentic state in question. You may well need to continue working on it for some time. As it is likely that your maladaptive way of expression has developed over quite a few years, it is clearly not realistic to expect it to be resolved in just a few minutes. However, if you do the exercise on a regular basis, coupled with the next activity, you are likely to see some results fairly quickly, however small they may be initially.

Activity

Again, begin by centring up to the point where you are in a state of all-round awareness. Next, focus on the area of your body where your chosen sentic state is located, and again say the word slowly six or seven times in your mind. Then begin to breathe a little deeper and with each breath imagine that you are breathing positive energy into the area in your body, and breathing out negative energy. Some people find it helpful to visualise positive energy as golden sunlight and negative energy as black smoke, but you may like to develop your own ways of doing this. After about five minutes, bring your attention back to the room as before, and, following the same procedure, open your eyes.

The above exercise is based on the premise that 'energy attracts like energy' and that 'what you put out is what you attract' (Jeffers

1992: 161, 83). Thus, the more you are able to comfortably express the various sentic states positively as a supervisor, the more you will help your supervisees to do the same. Below we give examples of how the various states can affect the supervisory process.

Awe

Here the aim is to be able to genuinely marvel at the good, the great and the unexpected, without feeling threatened or diminished. However, someone without a healthy sense of awe and with low self-esteem may express it by being incapacitated, and either be unable to act or slavishly follow someone perceived as a hero. In supervision, this is something to guard against. It is possible to get excited by whatever the supervisee is bringing and brilliantly analyse what is going on without giving him a chance to work it out for himself. Although they may initially be impressed, supervisees with a healthy sense of awe (as well as anger) will end up feeling frustrated. Others, however, may come to rely on the supervisor to always provide the answer, thus preventing themselves from growing and developing. They may be so in awe of the supervisor that they come close to idealising her and would never dream of challenging the situation.

Clearly, having a healthy, well-adjusted sense of awe is important to be an effective supervisor. Indeed someone with a complete lack of awe would find it difficult to act as supervisor, and would be unlikely to be chosen, as their cynicism and feelings of incompetence would stand in the way of positively helping someone to reflect on a work-related issue.

Joy

If joy is absent we feel down, depressed, lacking energy and our morale is low. Sounds familiar? It is my impression that many nurses feel like this at the moment, possibly not realising that 'what you put out is what you attract' (Jeffers 1992: 83). A depressed supervisor is an ineffective supervisor, and if this is you, you are in urgent need of injecting some joy into your life.

Supervision can be fun, indeed it can be great fun. It is all right to laugh, to play and to try out new ideas. Often the most effective people also have a well-developed sense of joy and playfulness, hence the expression 'work hard and play hard'. Ideally we would all work 'joyfully', finding pleasure, delight and fun in what we do. To be a supervisor who is a pleasure to be with, you need to enjoy what you do and be able to infect others with your enthusiasm and motivate them to grow and develop in their job. The enthusiasm does need to be focused, though. We have all probably met people who get excited quickly, but take on so many things that they literally are 'all over the place', never accomplishing very much.

The importance of the sentic state of joy is not to be underestimated and its appropriate expression is sorely needed in most areas where nurses work. Ultimately, people who work with joy are likely to contribute greatly to the quality of care and help provide an environment that is truly healing.

Eros

Unfortunately, there is something about a health care environment in general, and about hospitals in particular, that militates against the sentic state of eros. People who lack eros tend to be rigid in their views and like strict routines. As they are out of touch with their own bodies, they are insensitive to the comfort of others. Menzies Lyth's observation a few decades ago, that nurses tend to keep a 'professional distance' which contributed little to patients' comfort and well-being, may be reframed as a lack of a sense of eros (Menzies Lyth 1988).

Opinions may vary as to what extent Menzies Lyth's findings still apply today. There certainly is an awareness that professional distance is unhelpful, as is evident from the large numbers of nurses interested in undertaking counselling courses. However, it is our guess that still, too often, nurses are not sufficiently in touch with what is really going on for patients, mainly because they have not been at the receiving end of an appropriate expression of eros themselves.

'Being in your body' is really the only way to be. It is a very curious fact that many of us tend to regard ourselves and others as 'disembodied minds', or minds on legs. In order to be an effective supervisor, however, we need much more than our minds. Paradoxically, the less we use our minds and the more we are able to work through what we experience in our bodies, the more helpful we are likely to be. The previous two activities may already have given you a sense of what is involved. Supervision, like nursing, is a holistic activity. It involves our minds, bodies and, as we will see shortly, our hearts.

Love

'All you need is love' sang the Beatles in the 1970s, and to a large extent they were right. An appropriate expression of the sentic state of love would make supervisees feel safe, held and cared for. Being accepted, warts and all, by the supervisor would help them to accept themselves. Rather than beating themselves over the head for mistakes and errors of judgements, they would simply accept what they had done and set about whatever remedies were appropriate. In other words, the sentic state of love provides an environment in which a supervisee can grow and develop. Also, being nurtured themselves, supervisees will be better able to nurture those they care for and work with.

Supervisors with a negative expression of love, however, possibly because of a lack of love in some area of their lives, may use the supervisory situation to make themselves feel better. This can take the form of 'doing too much' for the supervisee, seeing him between sessions, going beyond the call of duty or sorting out his problems for him. Such a supervisor is unlikely to be able to offer any criticism of the supervisee, in effect going about creating the supervisory equivalent of a spoilt child.

Another way in which maladaptive love may be expressed by a supervisor is by looking for love from the supervisee. This may take the form of not really focusing on whatever the supervisee is bringing but instead using it as a starting point for talking about herself. Supervisors who frequently end up by telling supervisees how brilliantly they coped in similar situations, or how they had a similar experience, only ten times worse than that of the supervisee, fall in this category.

A lack of expression of love, on the other hand, leads to an over-emphasis on reason and logic. This is, of course, what is often valued in the world today, which is still to a large extent a male world with male values, where reason counts and emotions are taboo. This is not to say that a certain amount of reason and logic is not helpful in supervision, but that an overemphasis on it to the exclusion of nurturing leads to a barren relationship. Such a supervisor is likely to make supervisees feel uncared for or even judged as incompetent, which is unlikely to lead to a successful working alliance.

Grief

The work of nurses is often difficult and emotionally disturbing. If supervisees work in an acute area or in terminal care, for example, the death of patients may be a normal part of their working life, which means that, in effect, they suffer multiple losses. Supervision offers a space where nurses can offload some of these stresses. Even if no particular problem exists, simply talking about a situation and allowing oneself to feel whatever emotions are associated with it, in a supportive environment, is in itself supportive and helpful.

Positive expression of the sentic state of grief allows supervisors for their part to be open to hearing the nurse's stress and distress. If a supervisor feels comfortable with allowing a supervisee to express difficult emotions, she will be experienced as helpful and nurturing. A supervisors whose expression of grief has been maladaptive, on the other hand, may either try to minimise the nurse's experience and gloss over it, or become overwhelmed and unable to be supportive. Supervisors lacking an expression of grief will be experienced as hard, as they are out of touch with the emotion and have no idea what is going on for the nurse.

Anger

Anger, as well as hate, are two emotions which at first sight may seem strange to regard as desirable. This is because in our society both have become almost totally identified with negative expression. However, as we stated earlier, every sentic state has a positive as well as a negative expression, and anger and hate are no different.

Positive expression of anger is essential for a supervisor to be able to own her authority. A supervisor out of touch with anger is unlikely to be able to function very effectively, as she may feel too unsure of herself to criticise or challenge the supervisee when required. Positive anger means that such criticism and challenge is supportive rather than destructive. It is possible for a supervisor's anger with others to leak out in the supervision process, causing her to be overly confrontative and critical. The supervisee will end up feeling diminished, depressed or unfairly treated and angry himself. Anger tends to be less tolerated for women than men, causing many women to be either out of touch with anger or for it to go underground, leading to victim-like and manipulative behaviour.

A supervisor not in touch with the expression of anger will have difficulty in claiming her authority. A group supervisor in this position may find it impossible to keep a handle on the process, causing the group to be ineffective, go off at a tangent, avoid difficult issues or use one of their members as a scapegoat. As a lack of anger results in a craving for security and safety, a supervisor lacking anger will be afraid to take risks, will avoid thorny situations and, while possibly being very supportive, will not be as effective as necessary. Supervisees may experience such a person as somewhat wishy washy and the process itself as bland.

Hate

For many people this may be the most difficult state of all to see positively. It is, however, crucial for a supervisor to cultivate a positive expression of hate as without it, she will be unable to set boundaries. She may, for example, not know how to end sessions appropriately, always ending up rushing around trying to make up for lost time. Positive hate is clean, clear and cuts like a knife. It differs from anger in that if you are angry you want something to change (transformative energy), whereas with hate you want it to die or to go away (cutting off or pushing away energy). At a workshop, Peter Hawkins was observed demonstrating this point by pretending to wring a chicken's neck. It must be done sharply and decisively or the chicken will suffer (Hawkins 1995).

People who have problems with hate have difficulty with endings, with throwing things away, with finishing projects or relationships. Procrastination and workaholism are typical – clearly not a good role model for supervisees. A supervisor in touch with the positive side of hate, however, will be very clear about her own boundaries, communicate them clearly and stick to them. Consequently, supervisees will know where they are with such a person, helping them to feel safe. Generally such supervisors will have a healthy feeling of self-worth and in the supervision session, function totally in the 'here and now', rather than the 'there and then'. Such supervisors are unlikely to tolerate endless 'isn't it awful? or 'listen to what others have done to me' sessions, instead, focusing on what the issue is and what needs to be done.

Combining states

A good supervisor will feel comfortable with positive expression of all the sentic states and will move freely from one to the other. Although we have set out each state separately, in practice they are integrated and rely on each other for full expression. Positive expression of anger, for example, is best when combined with positive expression of love. Peter Hawkins (1997) states that 'the supervisee needs to experience your anger as well as your hate', while at the same time experience 'being held'. If a supervisee experiences incisive challenge while being supported, he is more likely to accept the challenge rather than defend against it. Evaluation of the supervision process itself is likely to be more effective as, having experienced that confrontation or criticism need not be destructive, supervisees may feel more free to challenge the supervisor or to offer an honest evaluation. Also, they are more likely to incorporate supportive challenge into their own way of working.

Activity

At this point it may be good to stop and note your reaction to all this in your journal. Note any resistance or disagreement you may feel to any aspects. Often the areas where we feel the greatest resistance or emotional reaction can offer the most fruitful learning experiences. If you do not notice any resistance or strong feeling in yourself, stop and carry out the activity on pages 92–93, which may give you an indication of what is going on for you.

I am not asking you to accept all this material uncritically (which would be like a negative expression of awe), but to look at it, consider it, and see what happens. You may find that you begin to notice things about yourself as well as about other people that you had not paid conscious attention to before. You may find that you suddenly see people's behaviour in a new light, which is likely to affect how you react to them. If you do have these sorts of experiences, note them in your journal. It will be useful to read through them from time to time, as it will give you an indication of your own development as a supervisor.

CONCLUSION

Supervision is something we *do* and any preparation should therefore include a substantial amount of doing, which is reflected in the number of activities in this chapter. At the same time, supervision provides a space for us to reflect on *what* we do, *how* we do it and *why*. In other words, supervision involves a reflection on the nature of nursing and what it is – or could be – about. As such it seems part of a new way of looking at nursing, away from abstract theorising. It seems congruent that any preparation for supervision would therefore focus on the activity of reflection and on self-awareness and self-development.

In this chapter, I have therefore invited you to reflect on your reasons for wanting to become a supervisor, what the role means to you and what skills you possess or may need to develop. I also discussed some essential listening and communication skills, after which we focused on the importance of an appropriate use of emotion. Throughout the chapter, however, I have homed in on the person behind the role of supervisor, while indicating the relevance of this to the activity of supervision. This chapter forms the basis for Chapter 5, in which the development of supervisors is investigated in more detail.

REFERENCES

Benner P 1984 From novice to expert. Excellence and power in clinical nursing practice. Addison-Wesley, California
Clynes M 1977 Sentics, the touch of emotions. Doubleday: New York
Clynes M 1980 The communication of emotion: theory of Sentics. In Plutchik R, Kellerman H (eds) Emotion, theory, research and experience. Vol. 1: Theories of emotion. Academic Press, New York
Epstein M 1996 Thoughts without a thinker, psychotherapy from a Buddhist perspective. Duckworth, London
Hawkins P 1997 Private conversation. 11 July, Bath
Hawkins P, Shohet R 1989 Supervision in the helping professions. Open University Press, Buckingham
Jeffers S 1992 Dare to connect. How to create confidence, trust and loving relationships. Piatkus, London
Kurtz R 1990 Body-centered psychotherapy, the Hakomi method. Life Rhythm, Mendocino, CA
Long A, Chambers M 1996 Supervision in counselling: a channel for personal and professional change. Counselling, February: 50–54
Menzies Lyth, E E P 1988 The functioning of social systems as a defence against anxiety: a report on a study of the nursing service of a general hospital. In Menzies Lyth I. Containing anxiety in institutions. Free Association Books, London, p 43–85

5

A model of supervisory development

...it is grossly inadequate just to send them on a short supervisor training course and then expect them to function well as a supervisor. (Hawkins & Shohet 1989: 79)

If supervision is to become an integrated part of every nurse's professional life, it is essential that there is clarity on how to prepare people for the role of supervisor. Benner (1984) suggests that in the course of their career, nurses progress from novice to expert. I suggest that supervisory development follows a similar trajectory and propose the Double Helix Model of Supervisory Development as a useful framework. The Double Helix Model comprises four developmental stages, each stage building on the knowledge, experience and skills of the previous level.

In this chapter, I discuss how people may progress from absolute beginners to experts in supervision. Characteristics and learning points for each stage of the model are discussed, augmented by a self-assessment questionnaire, which will enable people to gauge where they are in their supervisory development. As in Chapters 3 and 4, the style is interactive and contains activities, and I recommend therefore that reactions to the material are noted in a personal journal.

THE MODEL

Figure 5.1 shows the Double Helix Model of Supervisory Development, according to which supervisory development passes through the stages: novice, learner or advanced beginner, competent worker and expert. At first sight, the model may appear similar to Benner's model of professional nursing development. However, according to Benner's model, a nurse passes through five stages from beginner to expert, whereas the Double Helix Model includes only four stages. Unlike Benner, I do not split the final stage of mature adult/master into two stages of proficient worker and expert. This is partly because work carried out by others on supervisory development generally recognises three or four stages only (Hess 1986, 1987, Stoltenberg & Delworth 1987, Rodenhauser 1994, Watkins 1990, 1993, 1995).

More importantly, however, rather than regarding people at the expert stage as having reached some final summit of expertise, I see this stage as reflecting the inherently dynamic nature of working with people. According to this view, functioning as an expert involves the realisation that it is only possible to retain this level of expertise by continuing to practise as a supervisor, and to reflect upon that practice. Also, it means that learning never stops, as people are far too complex for any one person ever to be able to know, learn or experience everything that it is possible to know, learn or experience. The need for continued practice is recognised by the British Association for Counselling (BAC) who will only accredit supervisors for five years at a time, requiring evidence of a certain volume as well as standard of practice for reaccreditation. The BAC's policy is clearly based on the recognition that in order to remain at a certain level of expertise, continued practice is essential if one is not to decline in performance (Palmer & McMahon 1997).

THE PROCESS OF BECOMING A SUPERVISOR

The Double Helix Model provides a useful framework for conceptualising the process of becoming an experienced supervisor. The model is holistic and incorporates the development of appropriate skills, self-awareness and supervisory identity, as well as a knowledge of models, theories and an appreciation of the complexities of the actual process. 'I learn from every patient I nurse and every person I supervise', one supervisor said, indicating an understanding of how we learn from every encounter as each person and each situation is unique. For every stage of development the two strands of the double helix represent the characteristics of supervisors on the one hand and what they typically need to learn on

Characteristics
and skills

Learning
points

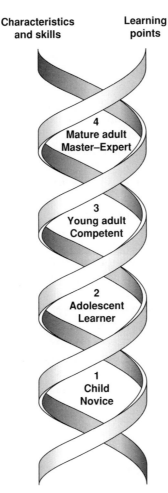

4
Mature adult
Master–Expert

3
Young adult
Competent

2
Adolescent
Learner

1
Child
Novice

Figure 5.1   The Double Helix Model of Supervisory Development.

the other. A self-awareness questionnaire and answers are provided in Appendices 1 and 2 which will enable people to gauge their own level of development in terms of the model.

The crossover points between the four stages mark the process of transition between each stage. Although for most people the developmental process is likely to be gradual rather than characterised by sudden spurts, each new stage will nevertheless 'feel' rather different from the previous one. In other words, clear distinctions can be seen between the four developmental stages, which is not to deny that development will also take place within each individual stage. Indeed, each stage is recognised as having its own areas of difficulty and crisis points, and for growth within (as well as between) individual stages to occur, a 'careful sequence of experience and reflection' is essential (Watkins 1993).

In other words, in order to progress up the developmental levels, it not only necessary to gain experience as a supervisor, but also to reflect on that experience. In congruence with the philosophies of reflection and supervision, I regard it as essential that such reflection is not done in isolation but under the guidance of a supervisor who is more experienced. In other words, in order to learn we need to sit at the foot of the 'master'. If we do not do so, it is hard to see how we can know what is involved in mastering the practice, and how we can know what it is like to be an expert.

Also, providing supervision can be a lonely experience if the supervisor does not have a forum for sharing ideas, problems and methodologies. As part of the process of becoming an expert supervisor, it is therefore useful to meet on a regular basis with other supervisors to compare notes and share experiences, guided by an expert supervisor. It is important to stress at this point that the emphasis here is on the support of the supervisor and the development of his role, not on the issues of his supervisees. However, as it is recognised that supervision is a good idea for all nurses, irrespective of their role or where they are working, some developing supervisors may choose to have individual supervision from an experienced supervisor, so they can discuss all aspects of their work, including supervision itself.

Reflection on supervision

In order to learn from their supervision experience I advocate that learner supervisors keep a journal in which to reflect on each session. Some people like to write in a 'stream of consciousness' everything that occurs to them about a session. Whereas this may serve a useful function as a memory aid, it needs to be accompanied by a structured reflection if learning is to occur. I therefore suggest the following format:

1. Identify the main issues from each session.
2. Write cameo descriptions of each main issue using What? Who? How? When? as guides.
3. Analyse the issues and identify themes.

The last activity is best done after a few days when it is possible to take a step back from the direct experience. It is also useful to take a block of journal entries, covering a number of sessions in order to see what themes emerge. Having identified the themes, ask yourself the questions:

4. What do I now know?
5. What do I now feel?
6. What am I left with?
7. What do I need to learn?

Keeping this type of reflective journal will aid in making unconscious knowledge and experience conscious, and will help to highlight areas of difficulty. It is a useful preparation for the supervisor's personal supervision or discussion with other supervisors, as it will help to ensure an effective use of time. Reflecting in this way also facilitates the development of an 'internal supervisor', by which I mean the habit of reflecting clearly, critically, honestly and dispassionately on everything we do (Casement 1985).

Activity

You will need thick felt tip pens or crayons and a large sheet of blank paper.

Imagine that you are asked to act as a supervisor to three people starting next week. How do you feel about this? How do you feel about your skills, abilities, preparation, etc? Portray how you feel, in whatever way you wish, using the felt tips and crayons. Before reading the next section, look at the picture you have produced and reflect on its meaning. What feelings are being expressed? If you can, discuss it with another person.

The activity of drawing pictures rather than writing things down is designed to help you get in touch with your feelings rather than with your thinking. It used to be thought that art work is associated with the 'right brain' which is involved with creativity, emotions and feelings, with the 'left brain' involving language and logical thought (Springer & Deutsch 1989). Whereas it is now believed that the explanation is more complex, it does seem to be the case that creative methods are more likely to help people get in touch with their emotions and feelings. According to Mollon (1997), this type of mental activity is not often taught at universities (where much of nurse education is now situated), not even in subjects that could clearly benefit from it such as psychology and medicine.

In fact, as we shall see when discussing the process of supervision, methods other than talking can be very useful aids to supervision. Apart from being fun to do, they also increase our capacity for finding alternative solutions to problems.

STAGE 1: THE NOVICE SUPERVISOR

Characteristics

Figure 5.2 sets out how, in my experience, people new to supervision tend to feel. To what extent does it concur with your position?

At this stage you are likely to be new to supervision and are unlikely to have received supervision yourself. Many nurses today find themselves in the position of being asked to act as supervisor with perhaps only a few days training. This is not necessarily a negative development, as we all have to start somewhere. However, it is important for employers to recognise that supervision is a skilled activity, which nurses cannot be expected to be expert at with only minimal preparation.

It is important therefore to support novice supervisors in their development and not to expect the impossible. Ideally, novice supervisors would receive close supervision on their supervisory role from an experienced person. Although there may not yet be many expert supervisors in the nursing world, they can be found in the professions of counselling, psychotherapy and social work. It may be useful therefore for nurses to look outside the nursing profession for such support if it is not otherwise available.

In a way, beginning to supervise with no or minimum preparation can feel like being a new student nurse all over again, a phenomenon sometimes referred to as role shock (Watkins 1993). As the role is new to them, people feel unsure of their own abilities, and indeed, are often unclear as to what exactly is expected of them. As a result, they may feel insecure and anxious which may be expressed in different ways. Some people will be open about their lack of experience and very hesitant to impose themselves too much on the process, letting the supervisee decide how the time is spent. In itself this is not a bad thing: being honest about your experience or lack of it will prevent supervisees from

Characteristics	Stage 1	Learning points
• Pressure to be seen to be competent (pretence at having more experience than is the case) • Possibly leading to authoritarianism (afraid to be 'found out' as incompetent) • Craving structure – as this is lacking without training • Role shock – insecure – unprepared – anxious • May have experience as supervisee – will use own experience as role model • No or very limited supervision training • Pressure to solve problem/give advice – do! before having 'heard' sufficiently • Uncertain re. purpose, function, goals, process • Tendency to stick to obvious facts only – concrete • Unaware of relevant knowledge and skills • Demanding rules, structure, 'this is how you do it' • Unwilling to challenge	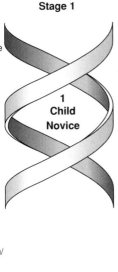 **1** **Child** **Novice**	• Relax – be honest about lack of experience – will reduce pressure to be expert • Ongoing training and feedback • Unlearn the 'having to do' nurse role • Further develop active listening skills – verbal and non-verbal, learn how to question effectively • Develop and learn to demonstrate qualities of empathy, congruence, non-judgemental (re. person – not what is done – normative) • Have supervision – to learn from being at receiving end – what works and what does not work • Identify strengths and weaknesses

Figure 5.2   Stage 1 of the Double Helix Model of Supervisory Development.

having false hopes and expectations. If it is paired, however, with an unwillingness to take on your share of the responsibility for the process, supervisees may feel that they are not getting much out of the supervision.

If, on the other hand, while being honest, novice supervisors are willing to have a go and share with supervisees what it is they are trying to do, this can work very well. Indeed, at some level, being relatively inexperienced can be an advantage, hence the truism 'it's good to be fifteen minutes ahead of your time, not fifteen years' (Wolff 1997). Supervisors who are very experienced can sometimes appear intimidating to supervisees, who may be reluctant to engage too much in the process for fear of looking stupid. Of course, supervisors should always guard against this but sometimes just having the reputation of being good and experienced is enough to intimidate others at first.

Sometimes new supervisors express their feelings of insecurity by appearing overconfident and authoritarian, as they are afraid to be 'found out' regarding their lack of knowledge and experience. They may feel that they are expected to be an expert and they revert to doing that role in the way such 'experts' have been with them. 'Never underestimate the insidious extent to which we are conditioned in the hierarchy in our culture' (Proctor 1996). Proctor was writing about counsellors learning to supervise, but her remarks about hierarchy and experts would seem also to apply to the nursing profession.

Pressure to solve problems

A very common theme among novice supervisors is the difficulty of listening to problems that supervisees may have without immediately suggesting possible solutions. One reason many people find this so difficult is that as nursing is often described as requiring a problem-solving approach, many nurses feel that it is expected of them to solve those problems. Also, nurses typically do things for people, in fact the modern nurse is often described as a 'knowledgeable doer' (UKCC 1986). Leaving aside for the moment whether nurses should always be solving problems or doing something, in supervision, it is inappropriate for a number of reasons.

First, if solutions are offered as soon as a problem becomes apparent, they are likely to be rejected out of hand. A typical interaction might involve the supervisor suggesting 'Have you thought of ...' or 'Why don't you ...', with the supervisee replying 'Yes, but ...' and then proceeding to give reasons why the supervisor's suggestions will not work. The supervisor may then suggest another solution, which will be equally rejected, and so on. Eventually the supervisor runs out of suggestions and the session has reached a stalemate, with both parties feeling very frustrated.

Why do supervisees behave in this way? Why do they not tend to take up offered solutions? The reason is timing. In many cases, solutions are offered before all aspects of the problem have been thoroughly investigated. It is therefore not surprising that they are rejected, as they are based on insufficient information.

The second reason is that often supervisees need to discharge their emotions regarding a problem before they are able to start thinking of possible solutions. They need to express their anger, frustration or sadness and for those feelings to be heard and recognised by the supervisor. The developmental work on sentic states discussed in Chapter 4 is particularly relevant here. There is no short cut. If people are not given the opportunity to express whatever strong emotions they are feeling, they will not have enough mental energy to apply to possible problem solving. Sometimes new supervisors are uncomfortable with this as they fear that the whole hour will be taken up with the supervisee complaining about some awful problem. Paradoxically, this is more likely to happen if the supervisee is not given the opportunity to express the emotion, as is the case when solutions are offered prematurely. In effect, this is what is happening, when the supervisee rejects the solutions saying, 'Yes ... but it will not work because ...' and goes on to express frustration, anger, or whatever she is feeling about the issue. In other words, she is saying to the supervisor 'you are not listening to me, here, I will tell you once again'.

A third reason why supervisees may reject solutions offered by the supervisor is that they may experience this as disempowering. Most nurses like to feel that they are in control of what they are doing, so it is better to guide supervisees to find their own solutions. Having been helped to generate their own problem-solving ideas, people are more likely to be committed to implementing them. After all, it is the supervisee who knows the reality of the situation; the supervisor only hears it second hand. This is where the skills of the supervisor really come in, helping and facilitating people to come to their own conclusions and make decisions regarding what is right for them in their own particular, unique situation, whatever that situation may be. Exactly how supervisors can do this is the subject of Chapter 6. Suffice it for now to say that the most important thing new supervisors need to learn at this stage is to relax, and not to feel the pressure to immediately solve everybody's problems. Relaxing by centring and using the listening skills discussed in Chapter 4 will be extremely helpful, and will encourage supervisees to thoroughly explore the problem or issue they have brought to the session.

The advantage of getting novice supervisors to relax and really listen to people, without the pressure of having to solve other people's problems, is that it gives them the freedom to think and to play with the material presented. Initially, this will seem strange to many nurses, used as they are to sticking to concrete facts and data only. However, in the field of interpersonal relations, whether it concerns interactions with patients, relatives or other members of a health care team, there are often many other factors that are not immediately obvious. Also, somehow it seems to be a fact of modern life that very few people will always say exactly what they mean. Thus most of us are in the perhaps rather odd position of having to listen behind people's words to the real message and, of course, often getting it wrong. It is this phenomenon that is at the heart of many communication problems. We often collude with each other in this facade, as simply speaking the truth about things can seem very threatening, either to ourselves or others.

Clearly such collusion would be unhelpful in supervision. In order to reflect, to solve problems, to achieve a 'super' vision, we need to work with the truth, not with some incomplete or sanitised version. By being honest and relaxed, supervisors can help supervisees to relax and be honest too, as the role of supervisor inevitably involves being a role model too.

The importance of experience

As far as novice supervisors are concerned, experience is needed before all this makes sense. Like nursing, the practice of supervision can only really be learnt in context. Whereas a certain amount of preparation is essential, people can only really learn by continually practising what they have learnt. Before progressing from novice to advanced beginner therefore, a certain amount of practice and experience is essential, as without it, any further material will not make sense. In other words, the development of knowledge about supervision and its practice go hand in hand. As novice supervisors are introduced to new skills and concepts, they need to practise these in order to integrate them with what has been learnt before. At this first stage of supervisory development, it is really important to practise the active listening and responding skills outlined in Chapter 4, and to focus on being honest as well as empathic.

Questioning

Learning how to question effectively is another very important skill, which often takes time and experience to develop. Most nurses know in theory that asking open rather than closed questions is more effective in getting people to talk. Yet in my experience most people find it very difficult. Especially when people first start supervising, they often bombard the supervisee with questions, most of them closed, with the result that the session quickly reaches a stalemate. When this happens a useful exercise is to try to conduct a supervision session without asking a single question, instead attempting to get the person to reflect only by using the skills of paraphrasing, reflection and summarising. Proctor (1996) calls the skills of clarifying, paraphrasing and reflecting 'the skills of empowerment'. I find that people are often amazed at how effective reflection can be in really moving people on, particularly if it is well focused.

Although there clearly is a role for questioning, I should like to stress that often, in this context, less means more. This is because if people are subjected to one question after another, they may feel that the conversation is turning into an interrogation, or that they are not really being listened to. The section below sets out some types of questions, as well as some dos and don'ts.

Types of questions

The best-known distinction involves open or closed questions, with the former inviting people to say more, and the latter only asking for specific information. Questions can, however, be further distinguished as can be seen below.

Closed questions. These may be used if all you require is a straight 'yes' or 'no' answer, or if you need specific information. They are, however, not helpful in facilitating reflection as they do not invite the supervisee to reflect.

Open questions. These questions cannot be answered by a simple 'yes' or 'no'. They may start with 'what', or 'how, or include a little preamble. It is not the case that questions starting with 'what' or 'why' are always open; for example, 'What time will you be off duty?' is closed, as is 'How many beds are there on your unit?'

Examples

- Open questions starting with 'what':
  - What were your reasons for deciding that particular course of action?
  - What other possibilities might there have been?

- What were your feelings at the time?
- What, I wonder, might this have meant for the other people who were there?

- Open questions starting with 'how':
  - How did that strike you?
  - How would you like to have acted?
  - How do you think you could do it differently next time?

- Open questions starting with a preamble:
  - I am curious to find out what went through your mind at the time.
  - I wonder what effect that might have?
  - You state that these changes are definitely going to happen, but what evidence, I wonder, do you have?

- Questions that invite the supervisee to enlarge on what she has been saying:
  - What else would you like to say about that?
  - Say a bit more about that?
  - Can you elaborate a bit on that?
  - What lies behind what you just said?

- Questions that help the supervisee to concretise and clarify:
  - What is it about that patient that worries you?
  - When you say that you did not feel yourself, what exactly do you mean?
  - It would be helpful if you could give a specific example.

- Questions aimed at uncovering people's personal thoughts, feelings and reactions:
  - How does that make you feel?
  - What are your thoughts on that?
  - I am wondering what the meaning of all this is to you?

Types of questioning to avoid

Asking too many questions. This may be experienced as interrogatory. Also, the supervisees may get in a habit of waiting for you to ask questions, rather than talking freely about what concerns them.

Asking more than one question at a time. This is very common. Often people tend to ask one question, immediately followed by another. This is very confusing for the supervisee who will generally only answer one of the questions.

Leading questions. These tend to put the answer into the supervisee's mouth, which may have several effects, all undersirable. The supervisee may go along with the answer, even if she does not really agree, as she feels that is what is expected. She may feel that you are not really listening or just do not understand, or you would not have asked such a question. She may even become angry or upset if she feels that you are seeing her in the wrong light. For example:

- Did you deliberately try to upset him?
- When did you stop reading the *Nursing Times*?
- You are not going to do that, are you?

Questions that are too probing, because they are too personal. These may have the effect of supervisees becoming anxious or resistant to exploring whatever it is you are talking about further. For example:

- How are you going to tell your husband about this?
- What effect is this going to have on your relationship?

These two questions are clearly too personal and do not fall within the remit of supervision.

Questions that are badly timed. For example, 'What did you contribute to that unfortunate situation?' when the supervisee is very distressed. If you feel that you really need to ask a question like this, it would be better to wait until the supervisee has calmed down and is thus in a better position to start thinking about it.

Questions that start with 'why'. These are best avoided as they have a tendency to sound critical or interrogatory. They may also remind people of the kind of questions they were continuously being asked by their parents or teachers, such as 'Why haven't you done your homework?' 'Why can't you behave in a responsible fashion?' or 'Why is your bedroom always in such a mess?' These questions are unlikely to have been helpful at the time, and they will definitely be unhelpful now.

STAGE 2: THE ADVANCED BEGINNER

Characteristics

Stage 2 is outlined in Figure 5.3. At this stage, you will already have a certain amount of experience as a supervisor and have received some training. The best scenario would be for you to

Characteristics

- Possibly having practised as supervisor – but without preparation – possibly leading to bad habits
- Some awareness of supervision theories and styles – as well as own skills, strengths and weaknesses – but tendency to over focus on weaknesses
- Fluctuating between over confidence and dependence
- Tendency to feel confused or feel lost in complexities
- Only vague awareness of impact of own style of relating
- Searching for a structure, model or theoretical approach
- Uncomfortable with challenge or confrontation
- Still a tendency to 'problem solve'
- Occasional lapses in objectivity
- Difficulty in maintaining boundaries
- Some tentative awareness of unconscious processes
- Impatient
- Didactic
- Wanting to seem clever
- Concerned with creating a good impression
- Either no probing or too invasive – unsure of balance

Stage 2

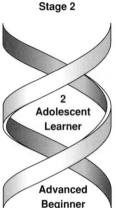

2
Adolescent
Learner

Advanced
Beginner

Learning points

- Unlearning possible unhelpful habits
- Develop an understanding of the process of supervision – both sessional and over. Learn to contract effectively and to evaluate honestly
- Develop more advanced skills – challenging, confrontation, focusing
- Learn to maintain boundaries
- Develop a consistently effective technique of note taking
- Gain theoretical knowledge and learn to begin to use in practice
- Become more comfortable with the release of difficult or painful emotions

Figure 5.3   Stage 2 of the Double Helix Model of Supervisory Development.

have ongoing training and support for your role as supervisor, as this will enable you to really learn from experience and help prevent bad habits from forming. If, however, you find that you are expected to function as an expert supervisor with only minimal preparation, I urge you to organise further training and support for yourself, possibly by means of supervision for your own supervision from someone who really is an expert. At present, many courses and study days focus on novice supervisors only, but as supervision is implemented more and more, there is clearly an increasing need for follow-up training. If this is not done, people are likely to stay at the stage of advanced beginner and clinical supervision will not be as effective as it could be.

The importance of structure

As well as being practised by individuals with the necessary qualities and skills, supervision needs to be practised according to a structure provided by an appropriate model. Which model is appropriate may depend on the area of nursing of the supervisee, as well as the personal preference of the supervisor. Novice supervisors generally find Johns' Reflective Cycle (see Chapter 1, pp. 13–14) easy to understand, although the way in which they use it tends to be limited by their lack of experience (Johns 1997). Nurses with a psychiatric background may like to practise supervision according to the Double Matrix Model, but as it is not very easy to understand without some experience, stage 2 may be a useful point at which to introduce this model (Hawkins & Shohet 1989) (see Chapter 1, pp. 10–19).

The model introduced in Chapter 6 takes the developmental stage of the supervisor into account, and is therefore a useful one for nurses to use from the beginning. Whichever structure or model supervisors have first been introduced to, at stage 2 in their development, it is useful for people to read about and experiment with some other ways of working, as this is likely to increase their repertoire of skills as well as their general understanding. Ultimately, people can only choose the way of working that is most effective for them if they have first investigated what is actually available.

Skills, strengths and weaknesses

In addition to a greater awareness of models other than those used so far, at stage 2, supervisors tend to be more conscious of their own skills and strengths, although there is a tendency to over-focus on things they are not yet so good at. Consequently, as is the case with many adolescents, stage 2 supervisors tend to fluctuate between feelings of overconfidence when a session has gone particularly well, and feelings of insecurity and a need for help when they feel out of their depth. Generally, people at this stage feel that they can function fairly well if a supervisee brings a straightforward issue which does not need too much reflection. However, when a situation is complicated they may be unable to see with enough clarity, and feel confused about how to help the supervisee, particularly if they still feel the need to solve all the supervisee's problems. A recent study carried out in Sweden, for example, found that supervisors often worried about their competence in situations of misunderstanding and felt a lack of self-esteem (Severinsson & Hallberg 1996).

I often advise supervisors, if they feel themselves getting lost or stuck, to stop and take stock of the situation by doing a summary as discussed in Chapter 4 (p. 85). For example, the supervisor might say: 'This is a complicated situation, let us stop for a moment and take stock of what we have talked about so far.' First of all this has the effect of providing both supervisor and supervisee with a breathing space, but secondly, and perhaps more importantly, the practice of summarising will itself help to clarify the situation. In fact, whenever you feel yourself getting lost, it is good practice to stop and not to go further until you are absolutely clear about what you have both talked about so far. Otherwise, progress is unlikely to be made.

Challenge and confrontation

Novice and advanced beginners in supervision are often very wary of challenge and confrontation as they are afraid that they may upset people. However, when potential supervisees are asked what qualities they would like a supervisor to have, they often mention someone who is non-judgemental while at the same time being able to offer constructive criticism. At first sight this may seem a contradiction in terms: how is it possible to be non-judgemental when criticism, however constructive, implies some kind of judging process? On probing a bit, it seems that what people mean when they say they want their supervisor to be non-judgemental is that they want to be accepted for who they are. Constructive criticism, on the other hand, they see as referring to what they do. In other words, people are in effect saying: 'Hey I'm an OK person and I would like you to acknowledge that, but obviously I am not perfect and sometimes I could do things differently; if so, please tell me'. This distinction between 'what I am' and 'what I do' is an important one to remember when there is a need to confront or challenge people.

Generally, a good way to challenge, confront or give constructive feedback is to 'wrap it up in a sandwich'; as one supervisee called it once, 'a sandwich made from lovely, fresh, wholemeal bread'. The bread stands for positive feedback, a recognition of what the supervisee is doing well, whereas the filling stands for the confrontation. In other words, people are much more likely to take on board a challenge or confrontation in a healthy way if at the same time they are recognised for what they do well – challenge works best if it is matched with support. Another reason for wrapping up a challenge in the brown bread of support is that it will help prevent people from beating themselves over the head for not being perfect. Many people, particularly women, have a tendency to focus on what they perceive as negative feedback, ignoring anything positive that is being said to them. By placing the challenge inside two positive messages, they are more likely to also hear the supportive feedback, thus making the overall message more balanced.

Conversely, receiving positive feedback can also be very challenging for some people. Some people are so unused to having supportive things said to them that they get suspicious and wonder what is behind the comment. Sometimes it seems that in our society it is more acceptable to put ourselves down than simply to accept what we do well. Also, when we are busy, as seems to be more or less the norm in nursing these days, it is easy to forget the niceties of life, such as telling people when they have done something really well, or thanking them for helping us out. Yet we all need to feel supported and appreciated in order to function well and feel good about ourselves. Therefore it is all the more important to get it right in supervision.

Boundaries

As a supervisor gets beyond the novice stage and becomes more effective at the process of supervision, he may feel a pressure to 'go beyond the call of duty'. Sometimes supervisees may be in need of such support that they want their supervisors to be available more than they have contracted for, or to be able to see them at very short notice when crises occur. However, supporting others begins with ensuring support for ourselves, and to be clear on what it is we can reasonably provide. If you have contracted therefore to meet once a month for an hour and a half, and your supervisee wants to see you every week, you need to be very clear about whether or not that is reasonable for you. Also, the request itself needs looking at. What is the reason for the supervisee feeling that she needs more supervision than originally agreed?

It is helpful to remember that every qualified nurse is an autonomous practitioner (at least as far as her or his own practice is concerned), and that supervision is not about propping people up, but about ensuring their professional standards and development in order to safeguard and improve patient care. Therefore, if a supervisee appears to have become rather dependent, the supervisor needs to ask himself what it is he has contributed to this situation. Somehow it seems that the more experienced the supervisors, the clearer they are about their own boundaries, and the less likely they are to engender dependency in their supervisees.

Another boundary issue is the actual topic being discussed. There can be a real temptation for supervisees to want to talk about personal issues, but this is clearly not within the remit of supervision. Again, it can be difficult for a supervisor at the advanced beginner stage to point this out to a supervisee, as it may feel like a rejection.

Clear contracting at the start of supervision (as discussed in Chapter 2) is helpful here as all the supervisor needs to do is to remind the supervisee of what they had agreed between them. If a supervisee persists in wanting to bring in personal material, it may be worth pointing this out to her and to suggest that she may need to find another forum for this. As supervisees are often confused regarding the difference between counselling and supervision, this is not uncommon, and it is therefore clearly the responsibility of the supervisor to maintain this boundary.

Unconscious processes

In any conversation there is always a great deal more going on than is immediately obvious. It is often stated that what is communicated non-verbally is usually more important than what is actually said overtly. Much of this non-verbal communication is within our awareness, or would be if we paid attention to it. There is, however, a third form of communication which is usually beyond our level of awareness. In other words, it is largely unconscious, yet capable of exerting a powerful influence on us. By giving careful attention to our own thoughts and feelings while listening to another person it is, however, possible to become aware of this form of communication. Often it can give a clue to important aspects of the topic being discussed which had hitherto eluded us. At stage 2 of their development, some supervisors may begin to develop an awareness of this form of communication, which is sometimes referred to as unconscious processes. Exactly what is meant by unconscious processes and how to work with them is discussed in Chapter 6.

STAGE 3: THE COMPETENT SUPERVISOR

Characteristics

At this stage (shown in Fig. 5.4) you are likely to have received a reasonable amount of training and are becoming quite experienced. You are continuing to have supervision for your own supervision and are committed to your own continued learning and development as a supervisor. Some people may regard you as an expert, but you know that there is still quite a way to go. However, you feel quite confident regarding what you can and cannot do. You have also developed your own style of supervising, although you are committed to continuing to learn new skills and models. Difficult and complicated situations no longer throw you off balance, as you have by now survived several of them. Naturally, it is always difficult to generalise; however, some supervisors, particularly women, may still feel uncomfortable with the practice of challenging at this stage, whereas men may actually challenge too much or too forcefully.

You understand the importance of self-monitoring and your 'internal supervisor' is therefore continuing to develop (Casement 1990). This means that you look to your own supervisor not so much for help and instruction as for consultative support and validation. The areas that you are likely to be really interested in and beginning to work with are in the field of unconscious processes, as you are beginning to realise the wealth of information this can provide.

Unconscious processes and their relevance to supervision will be discussed in detail in Chapter 6 (pp. 164–172), but for now, we mention that they include such concepts as transference, countertransference, parallel processes and projective identification. However, as we are all different, some people may at this stage

Characteristics

- Aware of own capabilities and style
- Possesses range of skills and experiences – to help with difficult situation
- More confident – although still tendency to occasionally down play own strengths
- Aware for a large part of the time of own impact on supervisees
- Able to work independently – developing a solid 'internal supervision' – using supervision consultatively – most of the time
- Becoming aware of more intractable 'blind spots' – seeking help in supervision to work with these
- Developing an identity as a supervisor
- Functioning at a more consistent level
- Aware of unconscious processes – although not always able to incorporate purposefully
- Perhaps still uncertain re. challenging (women) or overly challenging (men)
- Perhaps over focus on theory, analysis, cognition

Stage 3

3
Young adult
Competent

Learning points

- Consolidate the ability to balance the three functions of supervision
- Further develop ability to conceptualise (see the wood and the trees)
- Consolidate the skill of 'freely hovering attention'
- Develop ability to 'clearly bring a case' for supervision of own supervision – honestly stating areas of difficulty
- Become able to anticipate changes in supervisees' needs
- Consolidate the ability to use the 'here and now' – not just the 'there and then'
- Gain experience and confidence in using different methods (e.g. role play, visualisation, art work)
- Gain experience in working with supervisees from different backgrounds and cultures, races, genders, contexts, professional background
- Becoming 'good enough'

Figure 5.4 Stage 3 of the Double Helix Model of Supervisory Development.

not concern themselves too much with the unconscious processes relevant to supervision, but instead be (over)fascinated by clever theoretical analyses, which are mainly concerned with cognitive rather than emotional or unconscious factors.

The learning points for the competent supervisor therefore largely involve consolidation and further development of existing skills and knowledge. Gaining further experience by working with supervisees from different backgrounds would be very useful, as people's professional backgrounds and their culture, race and gender as well, as the context in which the supervision takes place, are all likely to provide unique learning experiences. The skill of conceptualisation, helping the supervisee separate the important from the peripheral and seeing a situation against the background of its larger context, is therefore an important one to build on at this stage.

As supervisors gain more experience, it is important to learn to vary their style of supervision to benefit supervisees accordingly. Whereas in the previous two stages supervisors may have felt the need to adhere to a fairly structured format regardless of the background or needs of individual supervisees, at this stage, it is important to learn to be much more flexible. Becoming experienced also carries its own dangers. It is possible to think, as soon as a supervisee starts to discuss an issue, 'Oh yes, I have heard this kind of thing before' and then not give the supervisee the attention that is needed. Sometimes it is possible to become so familiar with something that we forget that for the other person it is still completely new. Thus, what supervisors at this stage need to learn is the ability to retain their freshness in the knowledge that each and every supervisory session is new and unique and needs to be experienced as such, by the supervisor as well as the supervisee.

The three functions of supervision – normative, formative and restorative (or managerial, educational and supportive) – need to become more evenly balanced. Many supervisors do not find it too hard to be very supportive, but find the other two functions more difficult. The normative function includes the ability to confront supervisees if their practice is below par, which may be experienced as uncomfortable but clearly cannot be ignored. Also, at the earlier stages, the supervisor may not have felt sufficiently confident regarding the educational dimension and felt unsure how to go about things. Supervisors therefore need to learn facilitatory skills, that is, they need to develop the ability to help supervisees gain insight into the way they practise as well as how to go about remedying any deficiencies in either knowledge or skills. Although there clearly is a place for it, knowing when to impart straight information to a supervisee can be tricky as some supervisees can very quickly become dependent and expect the supervisor to always come up with the answers.

Scenario

Joan, an experienced supervisor, was becoming very frustrated with Sue, an E grade staff nurse on a gynaecological ward, who she had been supervising for 18 months. Although Sue had worked on the ward for a number of years, when problems occurred she rarely came up with possible solutions, which then led to Joan working very hard to think of ideas. In her own supervision, Joan reflected on this and said how angry she was beginning to feel and how she felt that she was really doing the work for both of them. Alison, her supervisor, helped her to look back on the history of her supervision with Joan in order to find out how this state of affairs had come about. Joan remembered that when Sue first came to her she was very newly qualified, very uncertain and seemed to lack much of the knowledge and skills that Joan felt she should have. Joan herself was fairly new to supervision at this point, and with hindsight, probably quite authoritative. She was so keen to let Sue benefit from all the knowledge she had that some supervision sessions almost ended up as teaching sessions. Sue was always very appreciative and frequently said how much she was learning from Joan. Alison, for her part, immediately realised what would be good to try, but she kept it to herself at first as she realised that in simply telling Joan she might create a similar situation between herself and Joan as existed between Joan and Sue.

She therefore modelled to Joan how to facilitate by asking her: 'What would you really like to say to Sue?'

Joan: 'I want to say to her, for goodness sake woman, you are an adult and a qualified nurse, start thinking for yourself for once'.

Alison: 'OK, and what else?'

Joan: 'Well I also want to say that I feel bad about it as it is partly my fault. I want to tell her that I have held her back by being too helpful but that we cannot go on like this any longer.'

Alison: 'You seem very clear about the situation. How do you feel you could discuss these things with her?'

Joan: 'Well, we have contracted for complete honesty in evaluations, but I for one have not been honest as I did not know how to say these things, and I guess I thought that if I am critical of her, she may be critical of me! I'll just have to bite the bullet. I know, I'll say something like we've been meeting for 18 months now, and as supervisory relationships tend to develop and change over time, it may be an idea for us to look at what has happened to our relationship. I don't think it has changed much, I feel we are stuck in a pattern, and I will say that, but it would be interesting to hear Sue's perception.

Alison: 'How honest do you feel you could be?'
Joan: 'Well, I know that if I want Sue to be honest and open, I will have to start with modelling that, won't I? Yes, I won't like it, but I feel it is the only way. I'll be honest with feeling frustrated, but own up to the fact that it is also partly my own doing. Actually, thinking about it, Sue probably thinks that the way we are doing it is the way it is supposed to be, I am the only supervisor she has ever had. I'll have to take most of the blame.'
Alison: 'Blame?'
Joan: 'Yes, OK, I know, I have a tendency to be too hard on myself.'
Alison: 'Yes, that is right. I think it is really good that you can see the situation for what it is, and your plan for dealing with it sounds as if it might work. But all that any of us can ever do is the best in the situation at the time. And I feel sure that is exactly what you have been doing, so the word 'blame' sounds a bit harsh. How would it be just to look at it as a necessary learning experience?'
Joan: 'Yes, that is helpful. I did not know any better at the time either. But now I do, so now is the time to do something about it.'
Alison: 'Good.'

In the above scenario, Alison skilfully allowed Joan to develop her own insight and solution while helping her to be realistic and positive rather than unduly punitive to herself. This she did by reminding Joan that all we can do is be as good as we can be in any situation. In fact, what supervisors need to learn is to be comfortable with being or becoming 'good enough'. Whereas self-monitoring by means of an 'internal supervisor' is an essential skill and habit to develop, it should not lead to destructive criticism. With hindsight, we will always see things that we could have done differently; however, in the situation we can only do what we can do – and that has to be good enough. A useful skill that will help with being good enough is that of free floating attention that I mentioned in Chapter 4 (pp. 81–84). Provided the supervisor continues to listen in this way, this skill will improve with experience and the potential information that may come to attention is likely to increase. Being in the here and now of the supervision session, rather than getting lost in the dynamics of whatever past situation is being talked about, is therefore very important.

What Joan, the supervisor, showed in the above scenario is the ability to very honestly and clearly bring an area of difficulty to her own supervisor. She actually needed very little prompting in coming to a conclusion, which is perhaps an indication of the excellent facilitation and role modelling she had received in her own supervision.

Another useful area of learning at this stage is to experiment with different media such as drawing, painting, visualisation or role play. However, as a general rule it is not advisable to try things out with a supervisee that you have not had experience of yourself. This is because first of all you may simply be unclear as to what to do or how to get the best out of it or, more dangerously, you may find yourself getting out of your depth. Alternative methods are fun, but if injudiciously used can occasionally have the effect of plunging people into painful personal issues which cannot be dealt with in supervision. Of course, it is inevitable that in supervision, people will occasionally find themselves suddenly in touch with some painful personal issue; as nurses work with ill and distressed people every day, this seems almost unavoidable. When it does happen, it is good to acknowledge it in order to decide what, if anything, the supervisee may need to do about it. In Chapter 6 (pp. 155–164), some concrete examples of a number of creative methods are provided, as well as ways of dealing with these types of unforeseen circumstances.

STAGE 4: THE PROFICIENT (MASTER) SUPERVISOR

Characteristics

At this stage (Fig. 5.5), you have 'mastered' the role of supervisor, are totally at home with the process and have consolidated your own way of working. You are comfortable not only with what you know, but also with what you do not know. Feeling confident in your ability to cope with any circumstance, you are nevertheless aware of the need to always continue learning and experiencing. Although relaxed about being seen by others as an expert, you realise the danger of over-identifying with this view of yourself as you know that every situation is different and that complacency is therefore to be avoided. You may therefore seek consultative supervision from someone with a different background and theoretical orientation from yours, as you see this as helping you to

Characteristics	Stage 4	Learning points

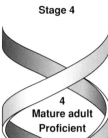

Characteristics

- Master supervision 'role mastery' – having 'mastered' the role process
- Has consolidated own theoretical position
- Confident in own abilities to provide good supervision and to cope with unforeseen, difficult and challenging situations
- Aware of need to remain open to new learning and experiences
- Knows that every supervisee, and every situation offers consolidation as well as new learning
- Seeks consultative supervision which is challenging and searching – possibly from someone with a different theoretical orientation
- Possibly training others, writing learning materials – articles about own experiences
- Comfortable with being seen as 'expert' yet aware of the dangers of complacency and rigidity. No need to appear 'all knowing and all seeing' – can admit to reflective lapses and errors
- Able to work competently with all levels of supervisee from a variety of occupation backgrounds, as well as different cultures
- Aware of and comfortable working with unconscious processes
- Able to draw on wide range of skills, experience, knowledge and to change gear and style smoothly as the occasion requires
- Able to function openly, honestly and non-defensively
- Comfortable with uncertainty and not knowing – realising the value of theory as well as its limitations
- Self-regulatory mature internal supervision
- Appropriate use of all sentic states
- Supervising other supervisors

Stage 4

**4
Mature adult
Proficient**

**Master
Expert**

Learning points

- Recognition of importance of ongoing learning development, reflection
- Mature internal supervisor
- Aware of – and comfortable with – not knowing everything
- Use a variety of methods
  – diary
  – art
  – role play
- Perhaps gain experience in different occupational areas
- To teach and develop novice supervisions
- To give talks about supervision – explaining purpose, concepts, process, benefits
- Learn to clearly articulate own way of working
- Further develop ability to smoothly move between sentic states

Figure 5.5 Stage 4 of the Double Helix Model of Supervisory Development.

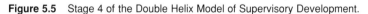

retain a fresh view of things and as being more likely to provide you with the challenge you need. You feel at home with unconscious processes and are able to utilise freely all the sentic states for the benefit of the supervision process (see Chapter 4, pp. 87–99).

You may have taken on the supervision of groups in addition to individual supervision and are probably being asked to teach and give talks about supervision on a regular basis. You may also be interested in developing your own learning materials and publishing articles based on your experience of supervision. Your internal supervisor is mature, yet you value your sense of playfulness which finds expression in your willingness to use a variety of creative methods, and a certain 'lightness' with which you carry your role.

Most importantly, however, you realise the essentially dynamic nature of being an expert, which means that you can only retain this level of expertise by continuing to practise supervision and to reflect on that practice.

CONCLUSION

In this chapter, I have introduced the Double Helix Model of Supervisory Development, which charts the progress of absolute beginners to the role of supervisor, via the stages of advanced beginner and competency to that of master supervisor. I have discussed the characteristic skills, knowledge and attitudes that people demonstrate at each stage as well as what they need to learn. A self-assessment questionnaire, which will give you an indication of your stage of development is included in Appendices 5.1 and 5.2. Having spent the last three chapters on how to prepare supervisees as well as supervisors, we are now in a position to turn our attention to what people actually do in supervision and how they do it. In Chapter 6, I therefore discuss the process of supervision in light of the Double Helix Model.

REFERENCES

Benner P 1984 From novice to expert. Excellence and power in clinical nursing practice. Addison-Wesley, Menlo Park, CA
Casement P 1985 On learning from the patient. Routledge, London
Casement P 1990 Further learning from the patient. Tavistock/Routledge, London
Hawkins P, Shohet R 1989 Supervision in the helping professions. Open University Press, Buckingham
Hess A K 1986 Growth in supervision: stages of supervisee and supervisor development. The Clinical Supervisor 4: 51–67
Hess A K 1987 Psychotherapy supervision: stages, Buber and a theory of relationship. Professional Psychology: Research and Practice 18: 251–259
Johns C 1997 Reflective practice and clinical supervision – part I: The reflective turn. European Nurse 2(2): 87–96

Mollon P 1997 Supervision as a space for thinking. In: Shipton G (ed) Supervision of psychotherapy and counselling. Open University Press, Philadelphia

Palmer S, McMahon G 1997 Handbook of counselling, 2nd edn. Routledge, London

Proctor B 1996 Supervision – competence, confidence, accountability. British Journal of Guidance and Counselling 22(3): 309–318

Rodenhauser P 1994 Toward a multidimensional model for psychotherapy supervision based on developmental stages. Journal of Psychotherapy Practice and Research 3: 1–15

Severinsson E I, Hallberg I R 1996 Clinical supervisors' views of their leadership role in the clinical supervision process within nursing care. Journal of Advanced Nursing 24: 151–161

Springer S P, Deutsch G 1989 Left brain, right brain. W H Freeman, New York

Stoltenberg C D, Delworth U 1987 Supervising counselors and therapists: a developmental approach. Jossey-Bass, San Francisco

UKCC 1986 Project 2000 – A new preparation for practice. United Kingdom Central Council, London

Watkins C E Jr 1990 Development of the psychotherapy supervisor. Psychotherapy 27: 553–560

Watkins C E Jr 1993 Development of the psychotherapy supervisor: concepts, assumptions, and hypotheses of the supervisor complexity model. American Journal of Psychotherapy 47(1): 58–74

Watkins C E Jr 1995 Psychotherapy supervisor development. Journal of Psychotherapy Practice and Research 4(2): 150–158

Wolff J 1997 The power of image. Brainstorm, the Creativity and Productivity Newsletter 17: 6

APPENDIX 5.1 SUPERVISORY DEVELOPMENT

SELF-ASSESSMENT QUESTIONNAIRE

Knowledge

1. How much supervision training have you had?
2. How much do you know about the purpose, function, goals and process of supervision?
3. How much do you know about theories and models?
4. How much do you know about different supervisory styles?
5. To what extent do you focus on theory?
6. To what extent do you focus on cognitive analysis?
7. Have you consolidated your theoretical position?
8. Do you know enough to teach others?

Skills

9. How easy is it for you to develop a supportive working alliance?
10. How often do you tend to stick to concrete facts only?
11. How much pressure do you feel to problem solve?
12. Can you negotiate a clear supervision contract?
13. Can you maintain boundaries of time?
14. Can you maintain boundaries of topic?
15. Can you handle complex issues?
16. How good are your active listening skills (paraphrasing, reflection, summarising, non-verbals)?

17. Can you use questions appropriately to help the reflection process?
18. How confident are you regarding challenge and confrontation while remaining supportive?
19. Can you help a supervisee to reframe a problem?
20. Do you get lost in the supervisee's issues and problems?
21. How good are you at getting the supervisee to focus?
22. How good are you at getting the supervisee to concretise?
23. Do you function consistently?
24. Do you balance the three functions of supervision (managerial, supportive, educative)?
25. How difficult do you find note keeping?

Attitudes
26. Do you feel pressured to appear as competent?
27. Do you have a tendency to be authoritarian?
28. Do you feel lost without structure?
29. Do you feel unprepared, insecure or anxious?
30. How confident do you feel?
31. Do you have a tendency to dominate?
32. Do you tend to feel a need to rescue the supervisee?
33. Do you tend to talk a great deal?
34. Do you seem to give a great deal of advice?
35. Can you acknowledge your strengths freely?
36. To what extent have you developed an identity as a supervisor?
37. How open are you personally to the need to continue learning?
38. How aware are you of the need to continue to add to experience?
39. What kind of supervision have you arranged for yourself?
40. Are you comfortable with being seen as an expert?
41. Do you feel the need to be 'all-knowing' and 'all-seeing'?
42. How comfortable are you with uncertainty and not knowing?
43. Do you find it difficult to be honest?
44. How open are you to constructive feedback:
    (a) from your supervisor?
    (b) from your supervisees?

Self-awareness
45. How aware are you of your relevant knowledge and skills?
46. How aware are you of your own strengths and weaknesses?
47. How aware are you of transference and counter-transference?
48. How aware are you of parallel processes?
49. How aware are you of projective identification?
50. How aware are you of your impact on supervisees?
51. How mature is your 'internal supervisor'?
52. What do you know about your blind spots?

Experience
53. Do you have experience as a supervisee?
54. How much experience do you have as a supervisor?
55. Do you have experience of supervising people from:
    (a) different specialties?
    (b) different disciplines?
    (c) different genders?
    (d) different cultures?
56. Are you considering writing about your experiences with supervision?

APPENDIX 5.2

THE DOUBLE HELIX MODEL OF SUPERVISORY DEVELOPMENT: ANSWERS TO SELF-ASSESSMENT QUESTIONNAIRE

Do your answers mostly fit column 1,2,3, or 4? Whichever column most of your answers fit will indicate your level of development

Stage 1 Knowledge	Stage 2 Knowledge	Stage 3 Knowledge	Stage 4 Knowledge
1 None or very little	1 Some	1 Recognised course, ongoing	1 Recognised course or equivalent
2 Nothing	2 A little	2 A great deal	2 What there is to know
3 Nothing	3 One model only	3 Have read about and tried working with several	3 As much as is available
4 Nothing	4 Some	4 Beginning to be aware	4 Have experimented with several, chosen own
5 Negative	5 Not much	5 Integrating it with own practice	5 Only as and when appropriate
6 Negative	6 Mainly	6 When appropriate	6 As and when appropriate
7 Negative	7 No	7 Beginning to have preferences but still learning	7 Yes
8 No	8 No	8 May be beginners	8 Yes
Skills	Skills	Skills	Skills
9 Negative	9 Can do it most of the time	9 Easy	9 Very easy
10 Always	10 Still a fair amount of the time	10 Not usually	10 Never
11 Over-whelming	11 Still quite a lot of pressure	11 Little	11 No pressure
12 No	12 Getting better	12 Yes	12 Yes
13 No	13 Most of the time	13 Yes	13 Yes

Skills		Skills		Skills		Skills	
14	No	14	Difficult at times	14	Yes, very occasionally unsure	14	Yes
15	No	15	Tend to get out of my depth	15	Most of the time	15	Yes
16	Unsure	16	Feel more confident	16	Good	16	Excellent
17	No	17	Much of the time	17	Yes	17	Yes
18	Not at all	18	Not confident	18	Confident most of the time	18	Very
19	No	19	Finding this difficult	19	Yes	19	Yes
20	Yes	20	Often	20	No	20	No
21	Not at all	21	Getting better	21	Yes, can do this nearly all the time	21	Very
22	Not at all	22	Tendency to forget this	22	Yes, can do this	22	Very
23	No	23	No	23	Yes, situation has to be very unusual to be off balance	23	Yes
24	No	24	Not really, one often dominates	24	Yes, as appropriate	24	Yes
25	Very	25	Difficult, tend to write too much	25	Note keeping now much more concise	25	Not at all difficult

Attitudes		Attitudes		Attitudes		Attitudes	
26	Yes	26	Yes	26	No, feel more relaxed	26	No
27	Yes	27	Sometimes	27	No	27	No
28	Totally	28	Yes	28	No	28	No
29	Yes	29	Often	29	No, feel well prepared	29	No
30	Not at all	30	Not very	30	Feel comfortable and confident	30	Very
31	Yes (or not at all)	31	Yes, occasionally	31	Have largely conquered this tendency	31	No
32	Yes	32	Yes	32	No	32	No
33	Yes	33	Yes, but getting better	33	No	33	No

Attitudes		Attitudes		Attitudes		Attitudes	
34	Yes	34	Yes, keep falling into this trap	34	No, only if appropriate	34	No
35	No	35	Sometimes	35	Yes	35	Yes
36	No	36	Not really	36	Yes	36	Totally
37	Very (or not at all)	37	Hope to soon know enough	37	Very	37	See it as crucial
38	Very	38	Very aware	38	Very aware	38	See it as crucial
39	Educative (role model)	39	Regular, facultative	39	Perhaps someone from a different background; an expert	39	Consultative
40	No	40	No	40	Not entirely, realise there is more to learn	40	Yes
41	No (sometimes yes)	41	Know it is not required, yet feel a pressure	41	Not really	41	No
42	Not at all	42	Not comfortable at all	42	Much more comfortable	42	Very
43	Difficult	43	Yes	43	No, not much	43	No
44a	Open	44a	It is getting easier to accept it	44a	Very open	44a	Completely
44b	Open	44b	Prefer to be told I am doing things well, constructive criticism from supervisee is difficult although helpful	44b	Very open	44b	Completely

Self-Awareness		Self-Awareness		Self-Awareness		Self-Awareness	
45	Not at all	45	Aware of some	45	Clear about what needs to be developed	45	Very
46	Not at all	46	Aware of some	46	Clear about own strengths and weaknesses	46	Very

Self-Awareness		Self-Awareness		Self-Awareness		Self-Awareness	
47	Not at all	47	Not really	47	Beginning to be aware	47	Very, although people may differ here depending on the preferred approach to supervision
48	Not at all	48	Sometimes	48	Much of the time	48	Very
49	Not at all	49	Not really	49	Beginning to be aware	49	Very, although people may differ here depending on the preferred approach to supervision
50	Not at all	50	Some awareness	50	Aware most of the time	50	Very
51	Non-existent	51	Quite immature and judging	51	Fairly mature	51	Mature
52	Nothing	52	Don't really know	52	Some inkling	52	Aware of existence, continuing to work on

Experience		Experience		Experience		Experience	
53	None or very little	53	Yes	53	Yes, ongoing	53	Yes
54	None or very little	54	Possibly one or two supervisees for a few months	54	A number of years	54	Many years
55(a)	Negative	55(a)	Hopefully yes	55(a)	Yes	55(a)	yes
55(b)	Negative	55(b)	No	55(b)	Beginning to	55(b)	Yes
55(c)	Negative	55(c)	Hopefully yes	55(c)	Yes	55(c)	Yes
55(d)	Negative	55(d)	Maybe	55(d)	Yes, or beginning to	55(d)	Yes
56	No	56	No	56	May be	56	Yes, probably, if not done so already

6

The Double Helix Model of Supervision

...the process of supervision is, by its very nature, fraught with potential paradoxes and built in conflicts which must be faced by both participants. (Baudry 1993: 597)

Intuition plays a large part in my life. (Newman 1986: 1)

'Is it always necessary to use a structure?' is a question novice supervisors tend to ask, as they often find it difficult to distinguish what happens in supervision from an ordinary conversation. The answer is 'yes' as without some kind of framework it is easy for the session to deteriorate into a general chat without any clear outcomes. The form of structure employed may vary depending on the needs of the supervisee and the experience and preference of the supervisor. In Chapter 1, various supervision models were discussed which may be used as a framework for the supervision process. However, with the exception of Johns' Reflective Cycle (pp. 13–14), these models were typically developed for the professions of counselling, psychotherapy and social work and may therefore only have limited application to nursing. The Double Helix Model of Supervision has been developed especially for nursing and takes into account the many and varied roles nurses undertake and the different settings in which they may find themselves.

In the previous chapter, we saw how the double helix provided a useful framework for the development of supervisors, with the creative tension between the forces of existing characteristics and learning needs combining to transform the novice supervisor into an expert, via the stages of advanced beginner and competence. Here, the framework of the double helix is used to help nurses navigate their way through the actual process of supervision. This chapter is in two parts: in the first, I discuss the model, followed in the second by a detailed discussion on what actually happens in supervision.

THE DOUBLE HELIX MODEL

The Double Helix Model was developed in order to explain the complete supervision picture and may therefore appear a little complicated at first glance. In this section, I therefore take you on a journey, explaining the model's construction step by step along the way. However, if you want to see the entire model before reading this section, it may be found on page 143 (Fig. 6.5).

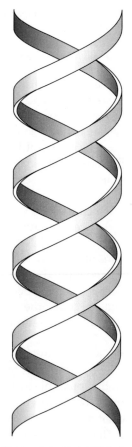

Figure. 6.1 A double helix.

Although I introduced the idea of a double helix in the previous chapter, it may be useful to start from the beginning, as some of you may have decided to read this chapter first. Figure 6.1 shows a double helix. As you can see, a helix is a strand curling upwards; a double helix is two curled strands, curling upwards together, giving the effect of meeting, separating, meeting, and so on. To me, the double helix very graphically portrays how clinical supervision involves not only the individual practitioner, but also the organisation within which the practitioner is employed.

Macro and micro

One strand of the double helix therefore represents the individuals within a supervisory relationship. I call this the micro level, whereas the other strand represents the organisation, or the macro level (see Fig. 6.2). To put it another way, by macro I mean the organisation or, if you like, the public arena that is there for all to see. By micro, on the other hand, I mean individuals' private worlds, which are not immediately accessible to others. So the macro world is the professional world, which is shared with everyone else in the organisation. However, whereas everyone who works for the same organisation shares the same macro environment, how that environment is experienced varies among individual nurses. This is because we all occupy slightly different positions, which means that our perspectives may vary as our experiences are never completely identical. Also, how we feel about an experience and make sense of it will be influenced by our personality as well as our own personal history. For example, if five people have attended a meeting, it is quite likely to have five different accounts of exactly what happened. That is because the macro world of the meeting gets integrated in the micro world of the individual, and as we are all different, that integration will be different too.

To summarise then, macro refers to the totality of the environment within which health care takes place, whereas micro refers to the individuals engaged in delivering that care. As is shown in Figure 6.2, the macro and micro sides of the helix meet and separate, meet and separate, almost like a continuous dance. In fact, I rather like the analogy of two dancers, elegantly moving towards each other, away from each other, towards each other, and so on. It seems that the dancers keep trying to go it alone, but find that they are irresistibly drawn to each other again and again, and are in fact in

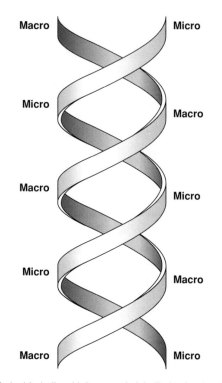

Figure. 6.2 A double helix with its strands labelled 'micro' and 'macro'.

a state of constant and delicious tension. Thus the macro and micro strands of the helix, like the organisation and the individuals within it, exist independently, but cannot do without each other. This tension is dynamic, because although macro and micro appear as opposites, both strands do inevitably influence one another.

For example, there may be tension between people at different levels of the organisation regarding what constitutes a good service. At an organisational level, there tends to be a drive towards ensuring a high-quality service with acceptable standards and a good level of efficiency and effectiveness. Individual nurses, however, may be primarily occupied with providing good care to the patients they are working with. So, although both the organisation and the individual nurse are in the health care business, there may be tension between them because the positions they occupy cause them to focus on different aspects, which can sometimes lead to conflict. Yet both positions are valid and necessary as the nurses cannot exist without the organisation and the organisation cannot exist without the nurses. In other words, they have to work together and use the tension between them to the best advantage.

Indeed, it would be a good thing for nurses to enter into a dialogue with the organisation and perhaps question some of the assumptions and decisions of the macro level. Equally, however, it would be good for the organisation to question the nurses, as such a two-way traffic would help to create a healthy environment within which to function, provided of course both sides are open to listening to each other.

As far as supervision is concerned, it is important to value both the macro and the micro strands, as both are essential to its success. Both the organisation and the individuals engaged in supervision need to be committed to its implementation, safeguarding and monitoring, although their reasons for doing so are likely to be different. However, this is part of the perhaps inevitable tension I talked about earlier. People at the macro and micro levels of the organisation are almost certainly going to have different views and priorities, but this is something we should work with rather than lament. This may seem difficult as the nursing culture has not traditionally valued opposites, conflict or resistance. Yet it could be argued that without conflict or difficulties to overcome there is unlikely to be progress as few of us would achieve anything like our potential without something to spur us on. Great personal tragedies, for example, may lead to tremendous personal transformation, provided the experience is worked through and digested, and we are prepared to learn and develop (Greenspan 1993: xxxix)

Clinical supervision is therefore neither about giving nurses a sop to ensure that they are good obedient workers who will not question the status quo, nor is it just about providing nurses with support and, metaphorically speaking, a shoulder to cry on. Clinical supervision is about helping nurses work through the everyday issues, conflicts or problems of their role and thus create a synthesis, an integration, or a greater vision of how best to exist within their working environment and, above all, how to ensure the best standard of care. Thus potentially every aspect of health care is there to be reflected on in supervision, not just the actual nurse – patient relationship.

It may well be that as a result of a supervision session, a nurse decides to tackle a problem by instigating a dialogue with people at the macro level of the organisation. For example, if staffing levels are really dangerously low, then supervision is not going to help nurses put up with that, as that would be in contravention of the UKCC Code of Conduct (United Kingdom Central Council for Nursing, Midwifery and Health Visiting 1992). Rather, nurses could use the supervision to reflect on what they can personally do to influence the situation, and how they might go about it, which will inevitably involve contact with the macro level.

What the above example makes clear is that modern nursing involves not only the care of patients, but also the safeguarding of the environment within which that care is taking place. In order to do so, it is necessary to have an agreed set of standards which are regularly monitored and modified in light of available evidence. Donabedian's (1969) standard-setting framework, incorporating the concepts of structure, process and outcome, has been very influential in nursing, perhaps because nurses realise that all three concepts are necessary. For example, structure refers to buildings and equipment as well as actual staff, process to what actually happens, and outcome speaks for itself. (This is a very short and incomplete explanation; if you would like to learn more about this approach to standard setting you may like to consult Parsley & Corrigan 1994.)

Not one but three

We started with the idea that clinical supervision involves a reflection on practice, and that nurses find it helpful to think in terms of structure, process and outcome. Also, as Bond & Holland (1998) point out, 'standards of care need to be at the root of clinical supervision' (p. 37). From here, it is only a small leap to incorporate these ideas in the model, by imagining three double helices, representing structure, process and outcome respectively. Figure 6.3 portrays the three helices separately for clarity. However, structure, process and outcome are intimately connected and cannot exist without one another. This means putting the three helices together in a single figure as in Figure 6.4.

The model as represented in Figure 6.4 may appear complicated at first glance. It may be helpful to visualise it as three-dimensional, and to imagine the helices in three different colours – say blue for structure, red for process and green for outcome – all gaily turning round in space, dancing in and out and connecting with each

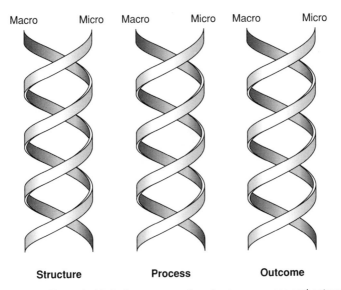

Macro   Micro   Macro   Micro   Macro   Micro

Structure   **Process**   **Outcome**

Figure. 6.3 Three double helices representing structure, process and outcome.

other at regular points. Each of the three double helices has a macro and a micro strand, so in effect we have a macro and micro strand for structure, a macro and micro strand for process and a macro and micro strand for outcome.

I will take each double helix in turn and discuss what this actually means in more detail. First, however, there is one final element that needs to be added to the model. Unlike many other clinical supervision models originating in counselling, psychotherapy or social work, the intention behind the Double Helix Model is for it to be firmly grounded in the nursing world. However, sometimes it seems to me that there is a lack of clarity regarding what nursing is. I have had many, sometimes very heated, discussions with groups of nurses on such questions as 'What is nursing?', or 'What is definitely not nursing', 'Are we a profession or perhaps a semi-profession?', 'Do we have an identifiable body of knowledge?', 'What is it we should be doing?', or 'What should we definitely not be doing?' and so on. As discussed in Chapter 1, this kind of debate has led to a plethora of nursing models and theories, all of which I see as part of our continuous growth and development as a profession. (Yes, I have decided to jump off the fence and call ourselves a profession for now.)

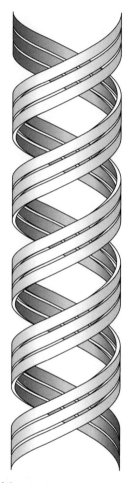

Figure. 6.4   Integration of the structure, process and outcome double helices.

I expressed above my wish to ground the Double Helix Model into the nursing world, from which it seems a short leap to incorporate an appropriate nursing model. I say appropriate, because not every nursing model is equally applicable to all areas of nursing. Also, whatever nursing model is chosen has to be compatible with the philosophy of clinical supervision. A nursing model that is applicable to all branches of nursing and which I think is also in line with clinical supervision was developed by Newman (1986). Newman's model is particularly elegant, and relatively simple to understand, which is a bonus. Obviously, it would not be a good idea at this stage to add an incredibly involved nursing model to the three double helices, as too much three-dimensional visualising may become too complex and offputting.

Basically, Newman's model consists of four concepts: (1) time; (2) space; (3) movement or change; and (4) consciousness. Newman sees these four concepts as influencing each other in a dynamic manner, which allows for continuous growth and development. She states:

We come into being from a state of potential consciousness, are bound in time, find our identity in space, and through movement learn the 'law' of the way things work and make choices that ultimately take us beyond space and time to a state of absolute consciousness. (Newman 1986: 46).

Time and space seem to be self-explanatory, and particularly relevant to nurses. Time is a precious commodity; we often perceive ourselves as not having enough of it. However, time is relative; if we enjoy what we do, time 'flies', whereas if occupied in something we dislike, the same amount of time may seem to last much longer. Equally, space is relative and closely linked with time. The enclosed space of a lift, for example, does not tend to go well with a long time, although it does depend very much on how the event is perceived by the individual. If being stuck in a lift for an hour prevents you from having to attend a meeting you want to avoid, you may be less upset than if you were about to meet someone you love. Equally, patients in hospital may experience the 'time' they spend on the 'space' of the ward very differently from the way it is experienced by a busy ward manager or a cleaner.

Movement or change refers to physical movement, such as walking, driving or moving house, as well as other activities such as work or perhaps recreation. According to Newman, we all integrate time, space and movement in our own unique way, which is at the same time an expression of our consciousness. Thus it follows that increased consciousness will have an effect on what we do (movement) as well as when and where we do it (time and space). For example, during the last few decades, with the growth and influence of feminism, there has been much consciousness raising, not only of women, but also of men, although some may argue that the latter has not gone far enough (Greenspan 1993). As a result of this change in their consciousness, many women have changed their way of life. Whereas before they may have spent all their time looking after their families (movement) in the home (space), now they seek work outside the home (space and movement) and continue their education (movement), all of which has had a great effect on how they spend their time. Equally, a period of serious illness (time and space), which in itself can severely restrict movement, often prompts people to ask questions such as 'Why me?, 'What is the meaning of this happening?', or even 'What is the meaning of my life?', all of which may lead to personal growth, or in other words, an increase in consciousness.

It seems that Newman's model fits the proposed view of clinical supervision perfectly, as I see it as a desire to continuously transform ourselves and our work through the increasing awareness brought about by reflection. In fact, the reason for choosing the double helix as the central concept of the model is because it stands for 'the eternal science of transformation' (Caduceus 1997: 5). Also, the strands of the double helix traditionally represent opposing forces which are believed to be in 'everyone and everything'. Examples of such opposing forces are 'activity and receptivity, light and dark, masculine and feminine' or macro and micro, which are believed to 'interact and create a spiralling process of increasing power (and) purpose' until integration is reached (Caduceus 1997: 5).

I see Newman's concepts of time and space as linked to the structure helix and consciousness to the process and outcome helices. Movement or change is relevant to all three helices as supervision is a dynamic process, and the way it is implemented at the macro and micro levels will develop continuously, leading to ever-changing outcomes.

In Figure 6.5, Newman's concepts of time, space, movement or change and consciousness have been integrated with the three double helices. Again, try to visualise the helices as moving or dancing in three-dimensional space, with the addition of each helix also exhibiting a continuous upward movement as indicated by the arrow. The latter is meant to show how Newman's concept of movement or change is integral to the model. In other words, the time spent in the 'reflective space' of clinical supervision results in continuous movement and change with the aim of increasing people's consciousness at both the organisational (macro) and the individual (micro) levels. As you can see, all the helices meet at regular intervals which I call *transition points*. In fact, I see the process of supervision as characterised by these transition points,

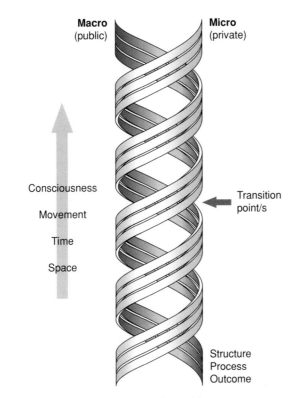

Figure. 6.5 The Double Helix Model of Supervision.

each of which indicates an insight or an increase in consciousness. Or to put it another way, each new increase in consciousness, which is in effect a new insight or a growth in 'super' vision, is an outcome of this process. I do not see this process, this movement and growth in consciousness, as ever stopping. This is because, as was pointed out in Chapter 5 (pp. 121, 124), without an openness to growth, there is stagnation and eventually deterioration. It is the recognition by the nursing profession of the need to continue learning and growing which has been a main impetus for the development of supervision. If supervision works well, this continuous transitional movement and growth in consciousness will occur at both the macro and the micro levels. In other words, individual practitioners will grow and develop but so will the organisation, leading to maintenance and enhancement of care at al levels.

Structure, process and outcome

Having put together the whole model, I will now discuss the helices of structure, process and outcome in more detail. As we saw above, the three double helices of the model, represented by the paired strands of structure, process and outcome, connect at the transition points (Fig. 6.5). However, although they make regular contact, each component denotes a different aspect of supervision. Although the helices of structure, process and outcome are interlinked and cannot really exist without each other, there is no linear or causal link between them (Donabedian 1969). So although a structure for supervision needs to exist in order for the process to occur which will then lead to outcomes, it would clearly not be possible to say that a particular structure would always lead to the same process, which in turn would guarantee certain outcomes. The reason why this is not possible is that we are dealing with human beings and not with machines. It is a fact that people, whether they are nurses, other health care workers, patients or relatives, are too different from each other to guarantee any similarity in outcomes. At the same time, as is the case with the setting of standards, outcome does depend on both process and structure, and process in turn needs a structure. So, let us have a look at each set of helices in more detail.

The structure helix

Macro strand. The macro strand in Figure 6.6 refers to the commitment by the organisation to supervision, in other words the structures put in place to implement it. This will involve such factors as premises, time given to staff for supervision, adequate staffing levels to enable people to leave their area for supervision, preparation of supervisors and supervisees and the system for bringing together supervisors and supervisees. Some of these factors may have financial implications, which means that ring fencing of adequate resources may be desirable. Structure also includes an agreed system of evaluation, both of its effectiveness and of the way in which it is being implemented, so straight away we can see how the structure helix and the evaluation helix exist without each other. Basically, the structure refers to the setting up and maintenance of supervision and all this involves, which means agreeing to abide by a contract between the organisation and the people engaged in supervision.

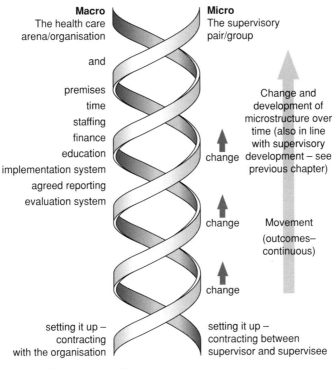

Macro
The health care
arena/organisation

and

premises
time
staffing
finance
education
implementation system
agreed reporting
evaluation system

setting it up –
contracting
with the organisation

Micro
The supervisory
pair/group

Change and
development of
microstructure over
time (also in line
with supervisory
change development – see
previous chapter)

change

Movement
(outcomes–
continuous)

change

setting it up –
contracting between
supervisor and supervisee

Figure. 6.6   The structure helix.

Micro strand. The factors of the macro level are reflected in the
micro strand. Thus people engaged in supervision need to have
access to suitable premises and be able to make use of the structures put in place by the organisation regarding time, staffing,
education and evaluation. In other words, the commitment to
supervision by the organisation has to be matched with a similar
commitment by individual practitioners. This commitment is
reflected in the contract between supervisor and supervisee, which
involves an agreement of what constitutes a safe physical and
emotional environment. Thus safety is characterised by boundaries
of when, where, what and how. 'When' refers to the time supervision is to take place, as well as its frequency and rules regarding
cancellation and rescheduling. 'Where' refers to the actual place,
whereas 'what' refers to clarity regarding what is and what is not
appropriate to be reflected upon. The process is referred to by the

'how', and involves an agreed way of working as well as the style of interaction between the participants in supervision. Examples of this are the preferred level of challenge, or the balance between the formative, normative and restorative components of supervision. A more detailed discussion of contracting may be found in Chapter 2.

Evaluation is relevant to the when and how as well as the what, and it is likely that over time there is change and development of both the macro and the micro aspects of structure in light of regular evaluation and achieved outcomes. Structure may also be affected by the preparation and experience of supervisors, and may therefore develop in line with supervisor development as discussed in Chapter 5.

Clearly the macro and micro aspects of the structure helix need to come together at regular intervals, as the people at both ends of the spectrum cannot do without each other. In my discussions with nurses, the point is often made that if clinical supervision is going to work it will necessitate a major rethink in how we organise ourselves and our time at both the macro and the micro levels. In other words, the implementation of supervision will involve the creation of protected time and space, in order to avoid the danger of it being sacrificed as soon as things get busy. For example, in many hospitals there is no longer the overlap between shifts that previously afforded time for teaching and staff development once the handover had been completed. Reinstatement of such an overlap would seem one way of creating time for clinical supervision, as in my experience, most nurses are opposed to supervision impinging on their own time. 'If we have to do supervision on our days off or add it to the length of our working day, it will add to our stress rather than help relieve it' is an often-voiced sentiment.

When I first started running workshops on clinical supervision in 1993, I found that nurses at lowers levels in the management hierarchy tended to be sceptical, indeed they were often antagonistic about the whole idea. They would voice comments such as 'Why are they doing this? What is it they are really after? I bet it is just a way to keep us in line or to get rid of us'. Equally, at the higher management levels there was often a similar misunderstanding regarding the philosophy of supervision, seeing it as an ideal tool to ensure that nurses did their job properly. Some years on, I find that nurses at both ends of spectrum have changed their thinking considerably. Although misapprehensions and misconceptions do still exist, many nurses now have a pretty good idea of what clinical supervision is.

What has changed is that nurses at the lower levels are beginning to say such things as 'We do not have to wait for management to implement supervision; there is no reason why we cannot make a start' or 'We need to make our views known to management or we may end up with a supervision system we are not happy with'. What also tends to come over strongly in my discussions with nurses is that many feel undervalued, which is not just a matter of inadequate salary levels. 'It is even more important to have better working conditions, adequate resources and decent levels of staff', they tell me. Nurses also say that they want the whole climate within which they work to be more humane and that more than anything else they want to be listened to, they want their point of view to be heard.

What I find encouraging is that nurses are also beginning to say 'If we want to be listened to, we have to make sure not only that we have something to say, but also that we do actually say it. We need to find out more about how the system works, who to talk to and how to go about making our views known'.

The outcome helix

The macro strand refers to the outcome of supervision for the organisation, whereas the micro strand is concerned with the outcomes of supervision at the level of the individual. As is the case with the structure helix, the two strands are interdependent, as outcomes from the micro level will feed into the macro level and vice versa (Fig. 6.7).

Micro strand. At a micro level, I see outcomes and the documentation of them afterwards, as part of every supervision session. In order to be clear about what has been achieved, it is good practice to set some time aside for this at the end of every session. Supervisors and supervisees may ask each other questions such as: 'How do we see what we talked about now?', 'What do we feel we have achieved?', 'What do we now know that we did not know before?', 'What new realisations do we now have?', 'What do I undertake to do between now and the next session?' and 'What new information do I need to seek?'.

Macro
(public)

Micro
(private)

Pooling of Micro
(periodical) outcomes

Independent measures
(to check whether
correlative changes
occur – e.g, sickness
absenteeism,
recruitment,
retention, complaints,
expressions of gratitude)

Evaluation of (e.g.)
every six sessions
re outcomes:

– formative
– normative
– restorative

Patient satisfaction
surveys

Other quality assurance
tools/measurements

Evaluation

Macro outcomes
pooled under:

– normative
– formative
– restorative

Evaluation of
every session

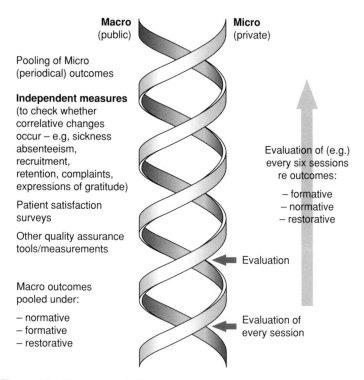

Figure. 6.7 The outcome helix.

So far, these questions focus on the actual content of the session, but it is also useful to focus on the actual process itself. So a supervisor may ask: 'How has this session been for you?', 'How useful has this been?', 'How did you feel I facilitated your reflection?' and 'What were you not happy with?', 'What would you like me to do differently next time?'. Equally, the supervisee may ask: 'How do you feel I engaged in the process?', 'To what extent do you feel I was open to looking at myself and my practice?', or 'What do you feel I need to do differently next time?'. Obviously it is important to be honest with each other and a good relationship is therefore essential. You may like to look again at Chapter 2 where the relationship between supervisors and supervisees is discussed in more detail.

The aim of focusing on the content as well as the process of supervision at the end of every session is to become very clear regarding exactly what it is that is being achieved. In terms of Newman's model, by giving ourselves the time and space to look at outcomes (movement), we achieve an increasingly clearer vision and greater consciousness, not only about the outcomes of what we have done, but also on how we have done it (Newman 1986). So the evaluation of clinical supervision at the micro level involves determining the outcomes of the 'what' as well as the 'how' of every session.

In addition to a mini-evaluation at the end of every session, it is good practice to contract for more formal evaluations on a regular basis. Some people like to carry out an evaluation every six sessions, which in the case of monthly supervision, works out as every six months. Obviously such an evaluation will become very much easier if both parties keep notes of the outcomes of individual sessions, as there is a limit to what people remember over time. In my experience, nurses are often surprised when they look back over their notes to find just what they have achieved. How the evaluation is done will depend on the individuals concerned as well as on what is required by the organisation. People often find it useful to group their outcomes together under the generally agreed functions of supervision, i.e. normative, formative and restorative (Proctor 1988).

Macro strand. At the organisational level, it is useful to pool together the outcomes from the micro level. For example, it would not be unreasonable to ask supervisees to provide the organisation with the outcomes of their supervision on, say, an annual basis. Obviously supervisees need to have complete freedom as to what they feel happy with divulging, but it could be along the lines of:

• Restorative: I feel less stressed now I have somewhere to talk about my practice.

• Formative: I have become more assertive and am therefore better able to function as an advocate for patients when necessary. I have also become a better communicator, both with staff and patients and find that I no longer shy away from talking to bereaved relatives.

• Normative: because of the way my skills have improved as outlined above, I feel my standard of care has improved. Patients seem to talk to me more and on several occasions they told me things they had not talked to anyone about, but which were nevertheless important and needed to be acted upon.

Of course this is only one example, and there are many other ways of doing this, but it does show that supervision can be evaluated directly by getting the information from supervisees themselves. In addition to pooling outcomes from the micro level, there is also a whole host of independent measures that have been mentioned as indicative of the success (or otherwise) of supervision. However, I just want to reiterate again that outcome cannot be divorced from structure and process. And, as stated above, although there is no linear connection between the three concepts, outcomes are unlikely to be positive if the structure is defective and people have been inadequately prepared for the process. Sometimes I find that because of limited budgets, managers are so concerned with wanting outcomes of supervision, that they begin trying to 'measure' its effectiveness without having invested adequately in its structure and process. In other words, unless there is a willingness to provide the resources regarding the structure (space, time, premises, etc.) as well as the process in terms of adequate training and preparation, there is little point in carrying out detailed outcome studies, as they would not provide a true picture of how supervision can and should function.

The process helix

The process of supervision as represented in Figure 6.8 is in fact the 'heart' of supervision as it is concerned with what actually happens in practice. Like the structure and outcome helices, the process helix is made up of a macro and a micro strand, both referring to the actual content of supervision sessions.

Macro strand. At this point, it would not be unreasonable to wonder what the macro strand of the organisation has to do with what is discussed in a session. Actually, a great deal. In an evaluation of supervision in England and Scotland, it was found that most supervision time was taken up with organisational and management issues (Butterworth et al 1997). Butterworth et al's findings are congruent with my own experience. I find that nurses frequently want to reflect on an organisational issue rather than on how they are working with a particular patient. Thus the organisation, in other words the macro environment, impinges on the supervision process via the topics that supervisees decide to bring. It seems therefore that supervision in the nursing world is

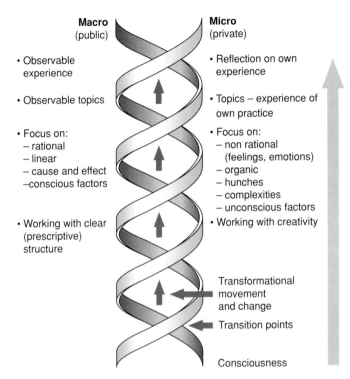

Figure. 6.8   The process helix.

different from how it is practised in counselling and psychotherapy, where the focus is typically on the client and what happens
in therapy sessions.

This may be because, as nurses, we are much more affected by
our environment than are counsellors and therapists. Equally,
whatever we do ultimately affects the well-being of others, either
directly or indirectly, and is therefore a legitimate focus for supervision. However, I postulate that there is more to it and that there
may be a link between a nurse's willingness to discuss her actual
nursing work with patients, the developmental stage reached by
the supervisor and the length of the actual supervisory relationship. This is because asking nurses to reflect on their practice in
the presence of another person is a relatively new phenomenon,
which is likely to feel threatening to many nurses. Unlike doctors,
who have always engaged in regular case discussions, we have

not traditionally been in the habit of inviting our colleagues to scrutinise our work. So in asking nurses to do so now, we are actually engaging in creating a shift in our culture towards openness rather than defensiveness and secrecy. Indeed, in this light, supervision is a logical development from the nursing process and its accompanying documentation.

As talking about our own practice is relatively new and may be experienced as threatening by many people, we need to feel comfortable and safe enough before doing so. Selecting our own supervisor and negotiating a working contract as discussed in Chapters 2 and 3 is part of creating such comfort and safety for ourselves. However, as was also discussed in Chapter 3, the development of any relationship takes time, and a supervisory relationship is no different. As the people concerned start to get to know and trust each other more, and as both become more familiar with the supervision situation, what is reflected on by the supervisee, as well as how it is reflected on, shifts from the organisational or public realm to the private. In other words, once a nurse feels safe enough with her supervisor she may be willing to reflect on aspects of her work that are closer to her personally. Equally, the more experience supervisors have, the more comfortable they will feel in the supervisory situation, and the more able and willing they may be to facilitate the process of shifting from the public to the private realm. Thus the actual process of supervision is always a dynamic interaction between supervisor and supervisee.

I have stated that it is not only a matter of what is reflected on, but also how that reflection happens that makes the difference between the macro and micro, or public and private, strands. It is, for example, possible to reflect on an organisational issue in a deeply personal way; equally, a nurse's work with a patient can also be reflected on in a superficial manner. Thus the distinction between public and private also involves the quality of the reflection. At the public level, our experience is observable by others and the chosen topic is more objective or engaged with in a less personal manner. The focus of the supervision tends to be on rational thought rather than feelings, emotions and intuitions, and frequently involves discussing the relationships between cause and effect. As stated earlier, people new to supervision often prefer to stay in the macro/public arena as it is less close to home and therefore less threatening. Another feature of people inexperienced in supervision is that they feel the need for a clear structure or model to guide them through the process (this was discussed in Chapter 5, pp. 106–110).

A problem with clear structures such as the Reflective Cycle (Johns 1997), or the Cyclical Model (page 8 Wosket 1994) is that nurses often have a tendency to use them in a prescriptive 'this is how you do it' way, possibly because it gives them a sense of security. In itself, this may be useful and form part of the developmental process as discussed previously. However, supervision should not get stuck at this fairly superficial level, which was of course never intended by either model. Another reason for the perceived need for a prescriptive structure may be the current focus on nursing as a rational activity which uses a problem-solving approach and is research and evidence based.

Micro strand. Looking at Figure 6.8, we observe that the macro and micro strands are interwoven and interconnected, to represent the fact that we need both rationality and intuition and that we need to reflect on both the public and the private aspects of our work. However, whichever level supervision is practised at, ultimately it is about helping supervisees to make sense of their experience in a creative and meaningful way. In order to help nurses free up their creative potential, it was therefore necessary to develop a model that is less likely to be taken as a blueprint. Basically, I see the model as a rough framework, as a space within which nurses can let go of some of their (sometimes self-imposed) restrictions and be creative. Newman (1986) has stressed the importance of space which, with time, is intricately linked with change and transformation, leading to greater consciousness of what we are about. Indeed, it is increased consciousness and self-awareness that are the focus of the micro strand.

Thus, in the micro or private sphere, we reflect not only on our care of patients, but also on how we use ourselves in every aspect of our work. So whereas in the macro strand the focus is on rational thought, as well as what is observable and objective, in the micro strand, we are concerned with the non-rational (to be distinguished from irrational), with feelings, emotions and intuitions, all of which are subjective and none of which can be directly observed. So in this part of the helix, we are not focused on cause and effect but are working with what may be unconscious, complex and organic, as it is a nurse's non-rational, intuitive abilities that distinguish the expert (Benner 1984). In order to access these non-rational abilities, the model therefore makes use of various creative methods, such as art, literature, poetry, music, sculpting, drama or visualisation, as they can help practitioners to free their intuitive potential and achieve a 'super' vision.

WHAT HAPPENS IN A SUPERVISION SESSION?

In this section, the process of supervision is discussed by means of scenarios and examples.

Preparing for a session

At the end of a session, Julie's supervisor Margaret said 'We got through a lot today'. 'That's because I want to get my money's worth,' Julie replied, 'and I do'. 'That may be so,' Margaret answered, 'but it is also because you have come prepared'. In fact all Julie had done was to write down the initials of the patients on whose care she wished to reflect, plus one or two sentences which to her encapsulated the essence of the situation. That is all she felt she needed as the rest was in her head; in all, it only took 15 minutes. However, Julie is in a habit of reflecting, keeps a reflective journal and makes good use of her 'internal supervisor' (Casement 1985). Thus for her, the actual preparation for a supervision session does not take much time at all.

In the same way that the discharge of a patient is said to begin at admission, the preparation for the next supervision session starts at the end of the previous one. Therefore, following a supervision session, it is good practice to jot down what actually happened, as otherwise it is easy to forget some potentially very useful insights. Julie, who sees her supervisor away from work and therefore has to drive home again after a session, finds it useful to record her thoughts immediately following the session into a little dictaphone which she always carries with her. That way, she says, she has logged what she finds useful and can write it out later when she has time.

Whether you choose to do the same as Julie and record your spoken thoughts first, or write down some key sentences, the important thing is that having done so, you are then free to focus on the next task that presents itself. This practice is particularly useful if your supervision is at the start (or in the middle) of your working day.

How to choose what to bring

In Chapter 2, (pp. 42–48) I discussed the importance of a contract between supervisor and supervisee so that there is agreement on boundaries and responsibilities. As the supervision is essentially for the supervisee (and through supervisees for the recipients of their care), many people feel that it should be supervisees' responsibility to decide which area of their practice they wish to look at. However, particularly when people are new to supervision and perhaps not used to reflecting on their practice, they may find this difficult. The following scenario is an example of how a supervisor can help.

Scenario

Cathy is an E grade staff nurse on a medical ward. She is supervised by Howard, a ward manager from the hospital's care of the elderly unit. They have met a few times to get to know each other and develop a contract. The first real supervision session was taken up with a specific problem that had occurred; this is the second session. Howard asked Cathy whether there was anything she needed to discuss regarding the last session and she said that there was not really, as the problem had now been resolved. She added that some of the ideas generated during the supervision had been very useful and had helped with the solving of the problem.

Howard: 'Good. So what would you like to talk about today?'
Cathy: 'I don't know, I haven't really got any problems at the moment.'
Howard: 'Well, supervision is not just about problems, but about how we work in general.'
Cathy: 'Yes I know that in theory, but I find it hard to think of anything.'
Howard: 'OK, let's try something. Think of yourself in your work area, see it as clearly as you can. You can close your eyes if you want to. Have you got it?'
Cathy: (Having closed her eyes.) 'Yes, I can see the nurses' station and a few of the single rooms.'
Howard: 'Now, imagine that you are walking around the whole area, having a good look round. Tell me what you see.'
Cathy: 'Well, I see the entrance with the ward clerk's desk. A little further on is the nurse's station and a bit further again

various other rooms. There's the doctors' office, the treatment room, the general therapy room.'

Howard: 'Mmmm, what else?'

Cathy: 'And there are the four-bedded wards. I can see some patients in their beds, some are calling out, but no one is coming.'

Howard: 'Can you see anyone else?'

Cathy: 'I can see a nurse sitting at the nurses' station, she is on the telephone.'

Howard: 'Anyone else?'

Cathy: 'Funny that, I can't see anyone, but they must be there, perhaps they are on break.'

Howard: 'OK, you can open your eyes now. What was it like to do this?'

Cathy: 'It's really strange that I could only see one nurse, that would never happen in reality.'

Howard: 'Perhaps it is how you feel sometimes? That you are on your own?'

Cathy: 'Funny you should say that, yes, I often feel like that. We are all so busy and at present we are three people understaffed because one person has left and has not yet been replaced, one has been ill for quite a while and one is on maternity leave.'

Howard: 'What is that like for you?'

Cathy: 'Well, I often feel that I am running around like a headless chicken, not really doing any one thing properly. I start one job, then remember another one, and am then probably called away to do a third. At the end of a day, I often feel that I have not given the quality of care that I should have.'

Howard: 'I am wondering whether it might be useful to use the rest of the hour to discuss how you could be most effective under the circumstances.'

Cathy: 'Yes, that would be good. I have been feeling for a while that I could organise things differently, without really being clear how.'

Howard then asked Cathy to describe a typical working day, and together they developed strategies for Cathy to try out. They agreed that Cathy would keep a diary in which she would outline how her shift was spent, what strategies she had employed to organise her workload and how effective this had been. They also agreed that she would create an agenda from this, selecting a few issues to talk about and prioritising them in order of importance to her. Cathy did, however, retain the freedom to postpone this to a later session if something more urgent cropped up.

The technique employed by Howard of getting Cathy to visualise herself being in her work area is a useful one. In this case, it helped the supervisee to focus on something that needed attention, but which she had not really let herself been properly aware of before. As an experienced supervisor, Howard knew that Cathy saying that she could not think of anything to discuss was probably due to her inexperience of supervision and not really being clear enough about how to go about selecting something. It is also possible, however, that a professed inability to choose what to reflect on, or a claim that 'because everything is fine at the moment, there is nothing to discuss', is a defence against something. In Cathy's case, for example, she had not really let herself realise that she was being ineffective, instead blaming it on being short staffed. So in a way she was being defensive. However, with Howard's help she realised that while perhaps not being in a position to remedy the staffing situation, she could take steps to work more effectively herself.

Both macro and micro elements are evident in the scenario, the macro being represented by the staffing situation, the micro by how Cathy herself was being affected. Cathy beginning to make changes in her way of working represents the double helix's concept of movement, leading, hopefully, to an increase in consciousness as evidenced by an expanded view of her work.

There are other areas the two people in the above scenario could have focused on. For example, Howard was struck by the fact that Cathy did not mention patients initially. He thought of mentioning this to Cathy but decided that this might be regarded as a criticism and therefore too challenging at this very early stage in their relationship. More importantly, however, Howard felt that he wanted to focus on Cathy and get a feeling for what work was like for her, which he did by some gentle probing.

Another way in which Howard could have helped Cathy to focus on something to talk about was to say: 'Think of your work area and pick one item that you see there'. Let us assume that Cathy said 'the resuscitation trolley'. Howard could then have asked Cathy to describe herself in terms of the trolley. For example,

Cathy might have said: 'I am a trolley with two trays, normally covered with a white sheet. I stand in the corner by the nurses' station minding my own business. There are lots of things on my two shelves that people use in an emergency. What I am not happy about, though, is that I should be checked regularly, this is not always done, I think, because it is not always clear who is supposed to do it. As a result, things sometimes go missing and I feel bad when there is a cardiac arrest and whatever it is they need is not there.' Howard could then ask Cathy to stay in her role of resuscitation trolley and ask her questions. He might ask her 'How does that make you feel?' and Cathy might say 'It makes me feel angry; if I am important enough to do all this crucial work, surely I should be looked after and given whatever it is I need.'

Although this may seem strange at first, Cathy the resuscitation trolley could then be used to help her to reflect on whether this is how she feels as Cathy the nurse. Usually it is, as after all, it was Cathy who chose to be the trolley in the first place. If she had felt very happy and cared for in her job she would probably have chosen to be something else. With this type of method, it is important to ask people to say the first thing that comes into their mind and not to censure it. This and other methods which I will discuss help supervisees to find out what lies underneath their rational thinking, as it is in the non-rational parts of our minds that problems often lodge, which means that the solutions are also to be found there. Also, for supervisees to be able to talk about how they really feel in their work is part of the supportive function of supervision. As has been pointed out by several authors, institutional changes and pressures can seriously undermine the ability of individual workers to stay committed, and empathising with patients can become difficult (Halton 1995, Baillie 1996). Supervisors, however, can help by allowing practitioners to express their feelings of frustration and distress, and to get them to be clear on what it is reasonable for them to put up with. Thus people can be helped to set limits for themselves regarding the extent to which they can cope (Halton 1995).

The method can also be used to help a nurse to reflect on the care of an actual patient. For example, Howard could have said: 'Think of a patient', followed by 'Now be that patient'. Then he might have asked Cathy as the patient, questions about Cathy as the nurse, which again, might have led to some useful insights. Or Howard might have said: 'Tell me about a situation when you made a difference to a patient's outcome'. This might have led Cathy to reflect on a positive situation in order to tease out what it was that made a difference. Conversely (and more challenging), Cathy could have been asked to reflect on a situation where she feels she was unable to make a difference to a patient.

Particularly with a new supervisee, it may be useful to focus on the here and now of the supervision situation. So when Cathy said that she could not think of anything, this could also have been due to feelings of discomfort. One way in which Howard could have dealt with this is by asking: 'Tell me, what is having supervision like for you?' or 'I am wondering what it is like for you to be here and to be asked to talk about your practice?' An even more immediate way would be to ask 'How are you feeling as you are sitting here?'. These kinds of questions would help both Cathy and Howard to place on the table any fears, possible misconceptions or feelings of discomfort. They could then have a dialogue about this which would help with the creation of a working alliance (see Chapter 2, pp. 35–40).

Choosing how to reflect

As was discussed in Chapter 2 (p. 47), it is good for supervisees to take the responsibility for deciding what to reflect on. If more than one issue or situation is brought up for discussion, it is also useful for them to prioritise, so that whatever is most important gets dealt with. Some idea regarding the time needed for each one is also helpful, which will get easier as supervisees become more experienced.

However, having chosen what to reflect on is only the beginning. Most situations are complex and can be viewed in more than one way, or from a number of different angles. So which angle to take involves a choice, as does the method of reflection to use. If both sides are happy to do so, it is useful (and often fun) to contract for the use of whatever creative methods seem appropriate to either supervisor or supervisee. The following scenarios will provide examples both of different angles to take and of a variety of methods that can be used.

Scenario: seeing other people's point of view

Claire, a ward manager, said to her supervisor William that she wanted to discuss the management of change as she had a problem. She wanted to introduce a different way of working with a particular group of patients, but found that two of her staff were resistant to this idea.

William: 'I have found that the more evidence there is that things should be done differently, the more some people cling to old practice. People whose minds are closed find new ideas very threatening. Let's try a bit of role play.'

William asked Claire to play the role of the two nurses while he acted as Claire. The role play helped Claire to see that her staff experienced being asked to do things differently as an attack on their world view, and on how they felt things should be. She also realised that they found it difficult to divorce themselves from the status quo, as this made them feel safe, and that they saw the proposed change as a personal attack. Also, as William told her, some people have an 'all or nothing' or 'true or false' view of the world. This means that in their world, things are either right or wrong. Therefore, if change is proposed because, for example, the latest research indicates that a particular kind of treatment (e.g. of leg ulcers, of pressure areas, of people with hemiplegia, or of people with schizophrenia) is believed to be more effective, for them, that is like saying that what they have done before is wrong – and they are not having that, as that would totally devalue everything they had been doing up to now.

What such people need is not more research evidence to convince them of the 'rightness' of the new treatment, but an understanding of the progression of knowledge. 'Right' Claire said, 'so what I need to do is somehow get them to see that they have been doing a good job until now, but that if they continue in the same way, in light of our new knowledge, it will no longer be the best.' 'Yes, said William, 'that will probably work. What else might help?' 'Well,' said Claire, 'I suppose I'd better prepare them for the fact that this treatment is likely to be superseded too, otherwise I have to go through the same process again next time a new treatment is developed, only then it might be worse.' 'How are you thinking you might do that?' asked William. 'I don't know, I obviously need to teach them about knowledge development and so on, but I don't think they will be able to cope with that. I found it difficult myself to grasp it at first. I have to find a way that makes sense, perhaps by relating it to something in their everyday life.'

'Tell me a bit about them as people.' William said. 'Well, they are both in their mid-forties, one is married, one divorced but both have adolescent children. I think their family really comes first for both of them.' 'Hmm, perhaps there is your answer, how could you use that?' After throwing the ideas around for a bit, Claire decided that she would set aside one hour a week for teaching sessions to which all staff who were available could come. She would run the first few sessions, but after that, anyone who felt they had something they would like to discuss or teach would be invited to do so.

This way, the two nurses would not be singled out, and also Claire would not carry the burden alone as some of the other nurses were very bright and committed and would no doubt jump at the idea. 'How do we know what we know?' would be the topic for the first session, and Claire decided to get people to compare how they look after their children compared to their grandparents and parents as a way into the topic.

The above scenario is an example of how the supervisor does not provide the answers, as all the ideas came from Claire herself. However, by asking open questions, and especially by getting Claire to place herself in the other people's shoes, the supervisor very skilfully facilitated Claire to solve her own problem. In other words, by the use of role play, William had helped Claire to take a different angle, which helped her to see the situation differently and which eventually led to a solution. Reflecting on a situation from different angles is important and should not be omitted.

Another way in which William could have helped Claire take a different angle is by 'rapid writing'. This involves thinking yourself into the role of the person and then writing whatever comes into your mind without thinking about it and without stopping for a preset amount of time (say five or ten minutes). It can also be helpful to give the supervisees a few questions and ask them to answer those from the role of the other person. The rapid writing method is one that we can also employ by ourselves as a means of reflecting in our journal, for example.

A slight variation to the role play is to ask supervisees to play both themselves and the other person and to physically move chairs each time they swap roles. So in the above scenario, William could have drawn up an extra chair and then have asked Claire to engage in a dialogue between her and the other nurses, sitting in the other chair whenever she played the other nurses' role. This method is quite dynamic and can help enliven a supervision situation that is lacking energy. Another advantage is that the supervisor, not being engaged in the role play, can ask questions both of Claire in her own role and in that of the other nurses.

Yet another variation is for Claire to play herself and the supervisor to play the nurses. The advantage of this method is that the supervisor will get first-hand experience of Claire in her working role, and also gain an idea of what it is like to be at the receiving end of her communication, all of which is useful information to feed back. The closer the chosen method gets to Claire and how she functions, the more the focus of the supervision moves from the macro to the micro situation, and the more challenging (but also the more useful and enlightening) it is likely to be. Supervisors therefore need to use their skills and experience to decide which method seems the most appropriate, not forgetting of course that the supervisee also needs to have a say in this.

Reflecting on the situation

In the above scenario, William helped Claire to focus on the 'what' of the situation, looking at it from different angles. This is an important stage which should not be rushed. As mentioned in Chapter 5 (pp. 108–110), in my experience, people new to supervision often feel pressured by the supervisee to find a solution as soon as a situation has been presented. This is not surprising with nursing often referred to as a 'problem-solving activity' which means that in practice, nurses often feel that they have to provide answers when presented with a problem, but in supervision this approach is counterproductive. Looking for solutions before an issue has been thoroughly investigated would be premature; also, providing the solution is disempowering for supervisees and does not facilitate their learning and problem-solving skills.

Staying with the not knowing and resisting the pressure to act is therefore an important supervisory skill. To go back to the above scenario, William might have said: 'OK, let's reflect on the last conversation you had with your staff. Go back to the first five minutes, how did it begin?' Or William could say: 'Just concentrate on five minutes of the conversation that seemed really crucial: show me what happened'. When doing this, it is useful to ask the supervisee to describe the setting where the conversation took place, perhaps even by moving furniture around in the supervision room. It is also helpful to ask her to describe exactly what each person looked like. For example, William could have asked Claire to 'become each of the two nurses for a moment, show me exactly how they were sitting and what they were saying'.

We often know the answer to a problem somewhere inside ourselves, but we need help in order to find it. Recreating the actual situation in the supervision room by means of the above methods is very helpful with this, as not only does it make the situation more vivid for the supervisee and is a great memory aid, but it also brings it alive for the supervisor. In other words, supervisors can see for themselves what was happening. It does not appear to be necessary to do this for the whole of the interaction, as in my experience, the essence of any interaction is present in even the smallest part of it.

To be effective, supervisors need to help supervisees to become aware of the filter through which they see things. 'Filtering' is something we all do, as there is in any situation potentially too much information for us to process (van Ooijen & Charnock 1994). However, in re-enacting the situation, what has been screened out in the description often becomes potentially available. It is the task of the supervisor to notice what has perhaps been edited out and to help supervisees become aware of this, which may involve challenging any assumptions they are making.

Reflecting on the nurse

To a large extent, supervision is about reflecting on what the nurse did, how it was done and why, and what, if anything, could have been done differently. Supervisees often want to reflect on people, relationships or situations in which they feel stuck. Such stuckness is often due to 'either/or' thinking, which means that people reduce their options and cannot see a way out of a situation (Hawkins & Shohet 1989). For example, a nurse may say: 'Either I confront him with what he has done or I look for another job' or 'Either I do everything she asks, however unreasonable that may be, or I will be seen as incompetent'. It is the task of the supervisor to help the nurse to see that there are always a great many more options. It can be useful to say something like: 'Imagine that by magic you suddenly know an answer. If that were to happen, what would it be?' It may seem strange but this strategy often works. Or the supervisor may initiate a brainstorm, inviting the supervisee to think of six different ways of dealing with the situation. Having provided six strategies, the supervisee is then asked: 'OK, now think of two more but they have to be really outrageous', or 'what is the wildest or most inappropriate thing you could possibly do?' In this way, supervisees are freed from the either/or thinking and become more creative. Apart from being fun, it is often in the wildest, seemingly most inappropriate ideas that there may be a beginning of the answer.

A similar strategy involves drawing a spider, with the problem in the centre and eight possible solutions drawn alongside the spider's legs. Once eight legs have been drawn, draw in two more. This may seem absurd as spiders only have eight legs, but this is an absurd spider and the legs therefore have to represent wild or crazy solutions.

Unconscious processes

As mentioned in the previous chapter (p. 119), in any interaction, much actually goes on below the surface without us being consciously aware of it. However, these below the surface or unconscious processes can contain a wealth of information which may be very useful, particularly when problems occur. The main processes are projection, transference, counter-transference, parallel process and projective identification, each of which I will explain below.

Projection

Projection means acting towards someone as if they were someone else (Page & Wosket 1994: 102; Fig. 6.9). In other words, material from one person is projected onto someone else. Frequently the person whose material we project is ourselves as many of us have a tendency to split off things we do not like about ourselves and project them onto others (Shohet 1989: 70). Indeed, projection may be a cause of many problems that occur in interpersonal relationships. The scenario below shows how a supervisor can help a supervisee to become aware of projection.

Scenario

Gail was accusing Bob, one of the managers, of being authoritarian and arrogant. However, as she later came to realise, it was not really Bob who was authoritarian and arrogant but her. In other words, Gail had projected something she disliked about herself onto another person, thus effectively disowning it. Getting a supervisee to see something like this about herself obviously needs to be done carefully and tactfully, as a blunt confrontation is very likely to be met with extreme upset, rejection or possible retaliation. Simone, Gail's supervisor, suggested a role play with Gail playing Bob, the role of Gail being played by herself. By asking Gail, in her role of Bob, how she felt, Gail realised that she had been arrogant and authoritarian herself, which she found very painful. She was, however, mature enough to realise that Simone had done her a real favour and it strengthened their working alliance. 'I can rely on you not to beat about the bush,' Gail said, 'and I need that'.

Transference

Transference is a term which has its origin in psychoanalytic therapy and refers to a projection from client onto therapist (Fig. 6.10). In counselling supervision, the supervisor attends to the transference by listening carefully to everything the client is reported to have said or done, including any throw-away comments that relate to how the client experiences the counsellor. It is very likely that transference does not just happen in counselling situations, but

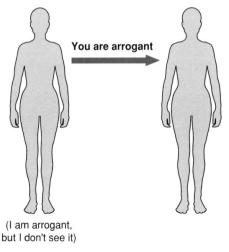

You are arrogant

(I am arrogant,
but I don't see it)

Figure. 6.9   Projection.

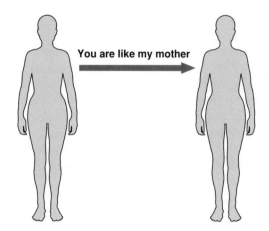

Figure. 6.10   Transference.

that we all project inappropriate material onto others all the time. This goes some way towards explaining the variations there may be in how the same person may be experienced by different people. Clearly, projection and transference may get in the way of effective communication and the ability to bring them to awareness is a useful supervisory skill.

Scenario

Jane had changed jobs as she had been very unhappy in her previous post. She had felt that her manager had criticised her unfairly, always finding fault no matter how hard she worked, and that she was deliberately kept in the dark about important decisions that were being made at the time. Her current manager, Mary, who also acted as her supervisor, was quite a different person, she was genuinely interested in her staff and keen to help them develop, which often prompted her to question her staff regarding what they were doing, in order to promote reflective practice. When Jane was asked to explain herself in this way, however, she reacted as if she were back in her previous job and became extremely upset, saying that if Mary did not trust her judgement and thought she was not good enough, she would hand in her notice that day. Clearly, Jane had projected her previous experience onto Mary; in other words, she had transferred material belonging to one person to another.

Mary was taken aback and became annoyed with Jane. Something did not feel right for her though and she took the issue to her own supervisor, who helped her to see that Jane's behaviour had seemed out of character and that transference was likely. Mary resolved to have a chat with Jane and to ask her to tell her about herself and her previous experience, something which she had meant to do anyway, but had not got round to. When she did so, all became clear and Jane and Mary were able to develop an honest and open working relationship, as Jane realised that Mary was truly interested in her professional development. However, the experience made them realise how difficult it is to combine a managerial responsibility with clinical supervision. They therefore agreed that it would be better for Jane to have a supervisor from a different area.

There are a number of strategies that supervisors can employ for finding out about transference between supervisees and others. Hawkins & Shohet (1989) suggest working with images and metaphors. In answer to being asked what would happen if she were alone with her ward sister on a desert island, for example, a nurse might say: 'I'd jump off and swim as fast as I could to get away from her', or 'I would build a shelter and do all the practical stuff while she sat around in a daze'. Clearly such an image provides useful information about the relationship between the nurse and her ward sister. It is also, again, playful and can be very therapeutic. It is important that the nurse says the first thing that comes into her head and does not edit anything out. Other useful questions suggested by Hawkins & Shohet include 'What animal does the person remind you of?', or 'What would a fly on the wall see looking at the two of you together?' Role play can also be used, with the nurse taking the role of the other person (or people) and being interviewed by the supervisor on their relationship with the nurse.

I find that instead of asking people to verbalise their answers, the above questions can also be answered by using art or poetry. For example, felt tips, crayons or paints can be used by getting people to portray their relationship with the person in whatever way comes to mind (Lett 1993). Alternatively, asking people to express their feelings in a poem can also be very effective, particularly if they focus on the essence of the relationship rather than whether or not the poem rhymes. In fact, modern poetry often does not rhyme at all, but when spoken, has a certain rhythm which can be very telling.

Counter-transference

Strictly speaking, counter-transference (Fig. 6.11) refers to the process whereby the supervisee unconsciously 'counters' any transference directed to her by the other person. For example, if a patient treats a nurse as if she were a forbidden authority figure, she may 'counter' this by going out of her way to be friendly and caring. However, it is also possible that she would behave uncharacteristically in an authoritarian way with this particular patient. As with transference, it is useful to bring counter-transference to conscious awareness in order to be clear about what is really going on in a relationship between nurse and patient (or others). Supervisors can watch out for counter-transference by paying attention to what is happening 'around the edges' of the supervisee's communications, such as images, slips of the tongue, metaphors or any non-verbal communications.

The term 'counter-transference' is also used to describe transference that is projected by the nurse onto the patient. Some useful strategies to bring this to light include asking 'Who does this person remind you of? followed by 'What is it you want to say to this person?' (Hawkins & Shohet 1989: 67). In this way, nurses are able to discover any unfinished business they may have with this person that is getting in the way of their relationship with the patient. It is then useful for the supervisor to ask the nurse to describe exactly how the patient is different from the person the

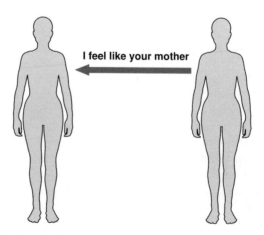

Figure. 6.11 Counter-transference.

nurse had transferred onto him or her, and perhaps for the nurse to role play what she would like to say to the patient.

The creative methods suggested for working with transference are equally effective with counter-transference. Indeed, art, literature and poetry are very helpful in getting people away from too much theorising and bringing them more in touch with their actual experience, thus greatly facilitating their continuous self-development and self-awareness (Lett 1993).

Parallel process

With parallel process, we use the 'here and now' of the supervision situation to reflect on the 'there and then' (Fig. 6.12). This is done by noticing how the supervisee is experienced in the session in the hope that this gives clues about how the supervisee really feels about the person under discussion.

Scenario

When Julie, a community psychiatric nurse, went to see her supervisor, Alan, she chose to talk about a new patient who she had not visited before. Normally Julie was well prepared for sessions,

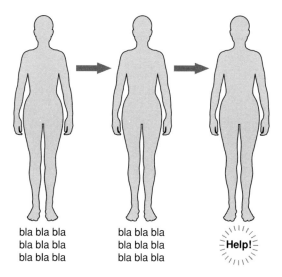

bla bla bla   bla bla bla
bla bla bla   bla bla bla
bla bla bla   bla bla bla   Help!

Figure. 6.12   Parallel process.

stating calmly what issues she was bringing and what she hoped to get out of the session. This time, however, Julie started talking as soon as she sat down and did not stop for ten minutes. Alan felt quite overwhelmed and tried to butt in a few times as he had trouble keeping up with her. Each time he tried this, however, Julie simply ignored him and continued talking. Finally, after ten minutes, Alan fairly forcefully asked Julie to stop as he was feeling totally lost. When he shared with Julie how overwhelmed, lost, indeed battered he felt, Julie burst out laughing. 'That is exactly how I felt when I was seeing this client,' she said, 'only I had not consciously realised it.'

Julie's behaviour is an example of parallel process, where supervisees unconsciously behave in the same way as the patient, in order to let the supervisor feel what they are feeling. It is important to recognise this phenomenon for what it is and not to get angry. If Alan had said: 'Julie, you obviously have not done your preparation as we agreed, I really cannot work with you in this way, it is against our contract', an important learning opportunity would have been missed. Also Julie would probably have become upset and the supervisory relationship might well have deteriorated. Instead, Alan acted 'subjectively', that is he responded from his own subjective experience in the here and now, and thus threw light on the there and then of the situation brought by the supervisee.

Projective identification

With projective identification, supervisors also use the here and now of the supervision situation (Fig. 6.13). However, whereas in parallel process the attention is on the supervisee, here supervisors focus on their own reactions and aim to notice any changes or shifts experienced in their own sensations and processes. Feelings that were not previously present, sudden images, words or phrases that somehow 'pop' into consciousness, are worth paying attention to, as they are likely to represent unconscious material that the supervisee is somehow transmitting to the supervisor.

Scenarios

Frankie normally looked forward to a session with Jack as they had built up a good working alliance. This time, however, she noticed that she was feeling unusually bored. She decided to test it out by saying: 'I notice that I am feeling bored at the moment, which I do not normally feel with you. I wonder whether that rings any bells with you regarding this particular patient?'

While supervising Richard, a nurse working in palliative care, Jill became aware of a strange sensation in her stomach, which felt like a great, empty hollow space. It was not that long since she had eaten lunch and therefore unlikely to be due to hunger. As an experienced supervisor Jill knew that feelings like this are often significant, so she said: 'I have no idea whether this is at all relevant to you, but as you are talking about this patient I am aware that I am feeling as if I have this great empty space in my stomach'. Richard, who had been talking about a terminally ill patient said: 'Gosh, that certainly does seem relevant. It is exactly what I feel and I think that it is probably how Dave, my patient feels although he is pretending to be fine and will not talk about his emotions'. Together the supervisor and supervisee then brainstormed how he might usefully help Dave to begin to deal with his feelings.

Projective identification can be very effective in group supervision as various group members often pick up different feelings, thus helping the person being supervised to see a more complete pic-

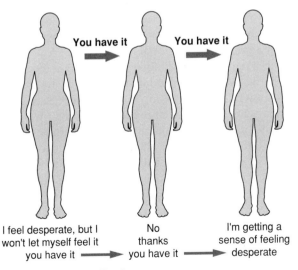

Figure. 6.13   Projective identification.

ture. This can work by asking the group to focus on their own feelings and bodily sensations while listening to the supervisee, rather than on the intricacies of the story.

As was discussed in Chapter 5 (p. 119), the more experienced supervisors become, the more they tend to focus on unconscious processes in addition to the more obvious conscious factors. Also, having been introduced to methods other than talking, many people enjoy the freedom and creativity they provide, as well as their potential for unearthing the less obvious factors. Thus they have the potential for greatly enhancing people's insight and learning, which in turn may lead to a more effective way of working. People also tend to find using creative methods therapeutic (as well as fun) which in itself adds to the supportive function of supervision.

CONCLUSION

In the first part of this chapter, I introduced the Double Helix Model of Supervision which has been developed specifically for the nursing profession and comprises the helices of structure, process and outcome. In the second part, I focused on the process helix and demonstrated how supervision cannot be seen in isolation, but is affected by the larger (macro) environment within which nurses work. The model is an ascending spiral, with each new insight precipitating a transition to a higher level of personal and professional development, a process that hopefully continues throughout a nurse's professional life.

The double nature of the helix also symbolises the fact that in supervision we work with duality, that is with the dark and the light, the knowing and not knowing, with successes and disappointments, with resistance and breakthroughs, in order to be continuously growing and transforming. Becoming aware of what is not immediately obvious, of what is in effect unconscious, is an important part of supervision and I have aimed to show how the unconscious can become conscious by the use of various creative methods. Between the not known and the known is the playful space of supervision, where we can reflect, dance, have fun, cry and be rejuvenated and encouraged, but also challenged in a loving, playful way. Supervision gives us a chance to look at ourselves, at the kind of practitioners we are, how we use ourselves in our practice, what we are doing and what we would like to be doing.

If we work in an organisation, we are all facets of a greater whole; we do make a difference. As we are part of the whole, we will have an effect, however small it may appear to be at the time. To the person it involves, an act of love is everything. It can be as small as getting someone a chair or a fresh jug of water. The important thing is that the other person will feel 'seen' by us, she will feel that she matters, that we see her as important. Nurses know that patients call for help, they call for healing, not only of their bodies, but perhaps even more of their spirit and their emotions. Being very ill is a devastating experience which shakes us profoundly and turns everything upside down and inside out. However, nurses can only continue to be with patients in their suffering if they are themselves also cared for. Thus supervision helps to counteract possible dehumanisation and depersonalisation, not only of us but also, and most importantly, of patients.

At a time when many of us seem to have to pack more and more into a working day, it is important to stand still from time to time, in order to rest, take stock and reflect on what it is we are doing. Supervision gives us an opportunity to do that.

REFERENCES

Baillie L 1996 A phenomenological study of the nature of empathy. Journal of Advanced Nursing 24: 1300–1308

Baudry F 1993 The personal dimension and management of the supervisory situation with special notes on the parallel process. Psychodynamic Quarterly 62: 588–614

Benner P 1984 From novice to expert. Excellence and power in clinical nursing practice. Addison-Wesley, Menlo Park, CA

Bond M, Holland S 1998 Skills of clinical supervision for nurses. Open University Press, Buckingham

Butterworth T, Carson J, White E, Jeacock J, Clements A, Bishop V 1997 It is good to talk. An evaluation study in England and Scotland. Clinical supervision and mentorship. School of Nursing, Midwifery and Health Visiting, University of Manchester

Casement P 1985 On learning from the patient. Routledge, London

Caduceus (1997) What is Caduceus? Caduceus, Issue 35: 5

Donabedian A 1969 Evaluating the quality of medical care. Millbank Memorial Fund Quarterly 4: 166–203

Greenspan M 1993 A new approach to women and therapy. Human Services Institute, Bradenton, FL

Halton W 1995 Institutional stress on providers in health and education. Psychodynamic Counselling. 1 (2): 187–198

Hawkins P, Shohet R 1989 Supervision in the helping professions. Open University Press, Buckingham

Johns C 1997 Reflective practice and clinical supervision. Part I: the reflective turn. European Nurse 2(2): 87–96

Lett W R 1993 Therapist creativity: the arts of supervision. The Arts in Psychotherapy 20: 371–386

Newman M A 1986 Health as expanding consciousness. Mosby, St Louis

Newman M A 1990 Newman's theory of health as praxis. Nursing Science Quarterly 3 (1): 37–41

Page S, Wosket V 1994 Supervising the counsellor. A cyclical model. Routledge, London

Parsley K, Corrigan P 1994 Quality improvement in nursing and healthcare. A practical approach. Chapman & Hall, London

Proctor B 1988 Supervision: a working alliance. Alexia, Sussex

Shohet R 1989 Dream sharing. A guide to understanding dreams by sharing and discussion. Aquarian Press, Wellingborough

United Kingdom Council for Nursing, Midwifery and Health Visiting, 1992 Code of conduct for the nurse, midwife and health visitor. UKCC London

van Ooijen E, Charnock A 1994 Sexuality and patient care. A guide for nurses and teachers. Chapman & Hall, London

Conclusion

In this book I have focused on the preparation of supervisees and supervisors as well as the process of supervision. Two models have been introduced: a model for the development of supervisors (Chapter 5) and a comprehensive model that encompasses the structure/implementation and the process as well as the evaluation of supervision (Chapter 6).

I hope that having worked your way through the book, you now have a pretty good idea of what clinical supervision is about. Sometimes clinical supervision is also called guided reflection. The interactive nature of Chapters 2–5, as well as the discussion of actual sessions in Chapter 6 demonstrate that reflection is at the very heart of supervision. Everything we do, from the mundane to the extraordinary, is worthy of reflection. In fact, clinical supervision can help us to see the extraordinary in even the most ordinary aspects of nursing.

Occasionally, it is necessary to look backwards in order to go forwards. This applies to reflection itself as well as the actual process of supervision. As was discussed in the chapters on supervisory development, sometimes new supervisors are so eager to be helpful that they do not give the actual reflection sufficient attention. Yet it is this reflection that constitutes the very heart of supervision. As was demonstrated in Chapter 6, the process of supervision can take many forms. I hope you will feel inspired to try some of the creative methods that were described, or indeed develop some of your own.

Supervision is not easy and we do ourselves disservice if we pretend that it is. Adequate training, of supervisees as well as supervisors, is therefore essential, as without it, clinical supervision is unlikely to be effective (Cutcliffe & Proctor 1998). As supervision is by definition something that is done with others, I have deliberately built in activities which have to be completed with at least one other person. The chapters on the development of supervisors and supervisees could therefore be used as a framework for a supervision training programme. As far as implementation is concerned, Chapter 2 will help those who start out with developing that all-important professional relationship. I know that many trusts are implementing clinical supervision and that some of them are developing their own training programme. I would, however, like to sound a note of caution. As mentioned earlier, unless people are adequately prepared and supported, clinical supervision may fail. It would therefore be better to go slowly but surely. The model of supervisory development discussed in Chapter 5 could be used as part of an ongoing programme of training and development. Ideally, I should like to see clinical supervision incorporated in pre-registration programmes, as the experience of receiving supervision is a very useful part of learning to become a supervisor.

As yet, there are not that many studies that clearly identify the outcomes of supervision. Sometimes people expect there to be a specific tool they can pick up and use to measure the outcomes of supervision. However, nursing is a complex activity and is carried out as part of a team. Any of the suggested benefits of supervision, such as increased patient satisfaction, fewer complaints and incidents, or improvements in the rates of retention, recruitment, sickness or morale, cannot be attributed solely to clinical supervision (United Kingdom Central Council for Nursing, Midwifery and Health Visiting 1996)

Perhaps the only direct method of evaluating clinical supervision is by asking individual nurses, as well as those working with them or being nursed by them, 'What differences can you see in them and their work?' By amalgamating such individual data, perhaps through existing instruments such as satisfaction surveys, professional portfolios or Individual Performance Review, it should be possible to build up a considerable body of evidence. The outcome section of the Double Helix Model may provide a useful heuristic for such evaluation (see Chapter 6). Indeed, preparing ourselves adequately, practising responsibly and auditing regularly is very much in the spirit of clinical governance (Department of Health 1998).

However, I would like to sound a note of caution. Over-reliance on outcome measures may result in losing sight of the process. Perhaps the desirability of supervision, if properly carried out, is self-evident. My hope is that eventually, involvement in clinical supervision will be regarded as an essential part of what it means to be a nurse. Perhaps we may even come to regard a lack of supervision as unethical. After all, if we do not support each other to reflect on our work, how will we know that we give good, or even excellent care?

REFERENCES

Cutcliffe J R, Proctor B 1998 An alternative training approach to clinical supervision: 1. British Journal of Nursing 7 (5): 280–285
Department of Health 1998 A first class service. Quality in the new NHS. DOH, London
United Kingdom Central Council for Nursing, Midwifery and Health Visiting 1996 Position statement on clinical supervision for nursing and health visiting. UKCC, London

Index